Medical Progress
and
Social Reality

SUNY series,
The Margins of Literature

Mihai I. Spariosu

Medical Progress and Social Reality

A Reader in Nineteenth-Century Medicine and Literature

Edited by
Lilian R. Furst

STATE UNIVERSITY OF NEW YORK PRESS

Published by
State University of New York Press, Albany

© 2000 State University of New York

For information, address the State University of New York Press,
90 State Street, Suite 700, Albany, NY 12207

Production by Kristin Milavec
Marketing by Anne M. Valentine

Library of Congress Cataloging-in-Publication Data

Medical progress and social reality : a reader in nineteenth-century medicine and
    literature / edited by Lilian R. Furst.
        p.   cm. — (SUNY series, the margins of literature)
    Includes bibliographical references and index.
    ISBN 0-7914-4803-7 (hc. : alk. paper) — ISBN 0-7914-4804-5 (pbk. : alk. paper)
    1. Medicine—Literary collections.   2. Medicine in literature.   I. Furst, Lilian R.
    II. Series.
    PN6071.M38 M39 2001
    809.3'9356—dc21   00-026534

10 9 8 7 6 5 4 3 2 1

To Ester Zago
dedicated teacher,
discriminating reader,
wise and encouraging friend

Contents

Preface

The aim of this anthology is to explore the literary portrayal of medical practice in the second half of the nineteenth century. The foundations of modern medicine were laid in the series of momentous discoveries and innovations that were initiated in the first third of the century and gained increasing momentum during subsequent decades. The introduction of the stethoscope, of anesthesia and asepsis in surgery, and the growth of an understanding of the way infectious diseases are transmitted are the foremost examples of the major advances made in the course of the century.

These advances have been amply documented in the many but often specialized histories of medicine that have proliferated in recent years as part of the expansion of the horizons of social history. However, much is to be gained by also approaching medical history through literary works because they offer a different, essentially personal, perspective. Literature reveals more fully than history the social realities in the dilemmas that physicians and patients alike faced in the wake of new discoveries and technologies. Through its focus on particular characters and situations literature affords vivid insights into the assimilation of, or resistances to, new modes of thought and new methods. So a vivid and nuanced picture emerges from literature of the directions in which the changing practice of medicine affected individual lives in many areas: in hospitals, in surgery, in medical training, in the rising role of laboratories, and in the advent of women doctors. Literature serves literally to flesh out medical history in crucial ways, particularly by revealing how erratic progress was in practice.

For while the history of medicine in the nineteenth century is generally presented, and rightly so, as a great march of scientific progress, the actual implementation of innovations proves a far more complicated process. Literary works are especially valuable for disclosing the variegated human responses to the scientific advances of the period. These responses run the whole gamut from enthusiastic embrace of the new to doubts, falterings, skepticism, and downright rejection. The picture of nineteenth-century medical practice that emerges from literature is thus a very mixed one: some practitioners and patients clung to the old ways, some made misguided attempts in partial ignorance to adopt innovations, some moved forward wisely and judiciously on the basis of sound knowledge, and still others were hampered from taking advantage of the benefits of scientific advances by circumstances such as lack of instruments or materials. This diversity of the social reality depicted in literature is a necessary corrective to the overly simple, optimistic assumption of an unchecked progression toward the conquest of disease. It is important to recognize instead the shortfall through both the slow cognitive acceptance of innovations and their tardy—and at times misguided—incorporation into routine practice.

I have chosen to focus on the second half of the nineteenth century because it is the time of the most fundamental changes through the transformation of medicine from a largely speculative endeavor into a discipline governed by scientific principles. The later nineteenth century unquestionably paves the way for present-day practice in salient ways (e.g., the ubiquity of the stethoscope as a basic tool), yet it still differs significantly not only in its technological possibilities but also in the issues faced by physicians, especially in the nature of the ethical dilemmas. To look at later-nineteenth-century practice is therefore, at least by inference, to realize the differences between the central problems facing doctors then and now.

The majority though not all the texts collected in this volume were written in the latter half of the nineteenth century. However, it is a mistake automatically to equate the date of publication with the timing of the action within the fiction. For instance, George Eliot's *Middlemarch*, which appeared in 1872, portrays conditions in 1829–1830; similarly, Thomas Mann's *Buddenbrooks*, published in 1901, chronicles the life of a family between 1835 and 1875, and Somerset Maugham's *Of Human Bondage* (1915) depicts medical training some twenty years earlier. Sinclair Lewis's *Arrowsmith* (1925), which opens in 1897 and extends into the second decade of the twentieth century, is included because it shows the full impact of laboratory discoveries on practice, albeit only at a temporal remove. Conversely, Mikhail Bulgakov's "The Steel Windpipe" (1916) illustrates the lingering therapeutic backwardness in a remote region where primitive methods still had to be used even in our century.

The first and the last selections are, unlike the others, not taken from literary works. To start with the Hippocratic Oath is logical because it continues to form the ethical basis of all medical practice. Its successors in the American Medical Association's 1847 *Code of Ethics* (and its 1980 *Principles of Medical Practice*) set the standards for the interaction of doctors and patients at their respective points in time. These documents define the ideal. By contrast, the last selection, Daniel W. Cathell's *Book on the Physician Himself* (1882) opens up an intriguing window onto the realities of the situation toward the end of the nineteenth century when an overproduction of physicians in the United States inevitably shaped the conduct especially of novice doctors toward their patients. These two sections together uncover the discrepancies and tensions between the ideal and the real, and so serve to enframe the quandaries depicted in the literary works.

Most of the texts I have excerpted are not otherwise easily accessible. Some (e.g., *Dr. Thorne, Middlemarch, Arrowsmith*, and *Buddenbrooks*) are very long, encompassing plots beyond medical interest. Others (e.g., *The Book on the Physician Himself*, the 1847 *Code of Ethics, The Mysteries of Paris*) are out of print. The majority of the writers chosen had medical connections of one kind or another. Several of them were themselves qualified physicians: Arthur Conan Doyle, Somerset Maugham, Daniel W. Cathell, and Mikhail Bulgakov. Others (Eugène Sue, Gustave Flaubert, and Sinclair Lewis) came from families with an extensive medical tradition. Still others such as George Eliot, Flaubert, Lewis, and Thomas Mann engaged in careful preparatory research to assure the accuracy of their portrayal of medical issues. Together the selections deal with England, France, Germany, and Russia as well as the United States. Although I am aware of the differences in the organization of medical practice in these countries and deal with them wherever appropriate, I am concerned here less with national distinctions and more with typological trends and tendencies.

This collection is not intended as a substitute for but rather as a complement to the study of medical history. The introduction provides an overview of the most important facets of medical progress in the nineteenth century, while the prefatory remarks contextualize each selection, explaining its significance. Finally, the list of further readings suggests possibilities for following up various topics covered in this volume.

I would like to express my gratitude for a Chapman Family Faculty Fellowship at the Institute for Arts and Humanities at the University of

North Carolina at Chapel Hill that gave me release time from teaching to work on this volume. I am indebted to Diane McKenzie of the Health Sciences Library of the University of North Carolina at Chapel Hill not only for help with information, especially about the development of instruments, but also for her supportive interest in the project. Without Janice H. Koelb's computer expertise in scanning texts and converting from one software to another, this volume would have been many more months in preparation; I am most grateful to her for her generosity with her time in performing this labor of love. My thanks go too to Susan Vida Grubisha, Gena Lewis, and William Nolan, my willing research assistants.

Introduction

From Speculation to Science

"Far more advances have occurred in medicine in the last hundred years than occurred in the previous two thousand," the physician-writer Michael Crichton asserted in 1970 in his book, *Five Patients* (New York: Knopf, 1970, 45). While agreeing with Crichton on the substantive issue of the immensity of the changes, medical historians see them as starting considerably earlier than he does. For instance, Charles E. Rosenberg, the foremost medical historian in the United States, maintains that "medical therapeutics changed remarkably little in the two millenia preceding 1800; by the end of the century, traditional therapeutics had altered fundamentally" (*Explaining Epidemics* [New York: Cambridge UP, 1992], 10). The French cultural historian Michel Foucault looks even further back: "Modern medicine has fixed its own date of birth as being in the last years of the eighteenth century" (*Birth of the Clinic*, xii). What is more, beyond the instruments, the diagnostic and surgical techniques, the remedies, and the growing understanding of the etiology and transmission of diseases, the changes also affected the entire underlying mode of perception: "Medicine did not simply become more scientific during the nineteenth century," medical historian John Harley Warner points out in *The Therapeutic Perspective* (7); "what was considered scientific, and what was not, changed." Empiricism, that is, faith in the primacy of observation, experience, and experimentation, ousted the old schematic, abstract system of a style of medicine sometimes called "library medicine" because of its pronounced theoretical orientation. One ready measure of the progress made by medicine is the doubling of life expectancy from 38 in 1830 to 70 in 1950, and to an average of 75.8 at birth in 1995 (white females 79.6; white males 73.4; black females 75.7; black males 67.9).

1

While such spectacular advances as open heart surgery, organ transplantations, and joint replacements have been in the limelight in recent decades, their foundations were laid in the basic scientific discoveries made gradually over the course of the nineteenth century. None of today's dramatic procedures would be possible without anesthesia, asepsis, not to mention that indispensable, ubiquitous instrument, the stethoscope, all of which originated in the nineteenth century.

The pace of progress was uneven. Occasionally something new appeared suddenly as when the French physician René-Théophile-Hyacinthe Laënnec (1781–1826), as if by inspiration though also by remembering the laws of physics, devised a stethoscope to meet the needs of a particular situation. More commonly success crowned long years of frustrating experimentation: the classic example is that of Paul Ehrlich (1854–1915) who, in 1909, synthesized a drug effective against venereal disease on his 606th attempt after 605 failures! Generally the process of innovation fell somewhere between these two extremes. So the stethoscope, though drawing on the same basic principle, was significantly modified from the 1819 version to its present form. Similarly, the ophthalmoscope, initiated in 1851, did not come into widespread use until 1880 after it had been simplified. Such protracted evolution points to a central problem in medical history: the difficulty of pinpointing precise dates. Sometimes crucial landmarks can be decisively fixed: rabies vaccine was produced in 1885, and diphtheria antitoxin in 1894. But when was the stethoscope incorporated into routine practice? The instrument was, according to travelers' reports, displayed in medical supply stores in Paris in the 1820s; however, it was not adopted even in the hospital of a large French provincial town, Clermont-Ferrand, before the 1850s. Unlike today, when information is rapidly spread through a host of biomedical journals (20,000 in 1981, and growing at 6 to 7 percent per year, doubling every ten to fifteen years), conferences, and the Internet, communications were slow and erratic in the nineteenth century. There was also a great discrepancy between the kind of elite, avant-garde medicine that became available in major medical centers such as Boston, New York, Philadelphia, Paris, London, and Edinburgh and the persistently primitive practices in remote rural areas (Flaubert, *Madame Bovary* [see "Surgery" in chapter 4], and Bulgakov, "The Steel Windpipe" [see chapter 8]). So medical history at some points allows the kind of definitive temporal markers that political history has in the year of a battle, the accession or death of a monarch; but more often it is akin to social history in tracing the gradual drift characteristic of changes in the fabric of society.

Humoral Medicine

Before the formation of a clear understanding of the workings of the human body in health and in sickness, medicine was predominantly speculative. Insight into bodily functions and disorders beneath the surface was very scant until the growth of anatomy. For example, the fact that blood circulated was grasped only about 1620 by William Harvey, a British physician who published in 1628 a Latin treatise, *De Motu Cordis* (On the Motion of the Heart), an anatomical study of the movement of the heart and blood in animals.

Lacking both sound knowledge and tools for probing examination, medical men had to rely solely on their senses by observing their patients and listening to the recital of their complaints. They would scrutinize their patients' appearance, looking at skin color, and paying attention to signs of wasting or bloating; they would feel the pulse to assess its rate and strength, and they would closely inspect the urine. Yet even the evaluation of this visible specimen would be largely guesswork, stemming at best from comparison with previous similar cases. The term "urinomancers" was coined to describe the approach of some medical men because they would invent diagnostic fables from the evidence of the urine. Patients' narratives of their symptoms were a central part of the transaction between doctor and patient, but they are potentially unreliable since they derive from exclusively subjective sensations, which may vary considerably from person to person, depending, among other factors, on tolerance for pain (pain threshold). Yet in the eighteenth century, confidence in patients' descriptions of their illness was so great that practice by mail was not uncommon, with doctors even forgoing personal observation in arriving at a diagnosis. While patients' narratives are the starting-point of medical consultations today too, they are immediately supplemented (and perhaps amended) by the results of objective, scientifically measured tests.

The cornerstone of medicine from the time of Galen, a Greek physician born in 130 A.D., was the theory of the four "humors." The universe was recognized as consisting of four elements: earth, air, water, and fire. These were taken to correspond in the human body to cold, dry, moist, and hot humors. It was thought that good health resulted from the right balance of the humors; when one or another got the upper hand, the proper corrective was to resort to its opposite, applying heat to cold areas and vice versa, and treating dryness and moisture as parallel counteragents. Certain bodily fluids were linked to particular qualities: blood was seen as hot and moist, phlegm cold and moist, yellow bile hot and dry, and black bile cold and dry. This doctrine was further extended to encompass a person's psychological profile, for it was believed that individuals were endowed with a preponderance of one humor or another, making them sanguine, phlegmatic, choleric, or melancholic, respectively.

In order to remediate the humoral imbalance regarded as the cause of disease, it was necessary first to establish the patient's distinctive humor. Then the chosen therapy was tailored to fit the particular patient in light of his or her dominant humor, age, and situation, that is, the time of year, the climate, the location, etc. Two patients with identical symptoms might be given wholly divergent treatments because of the perceived differences in their circumstances. So the outcome of humoral medicine was patient-specific treatment. This system runs utterly counter to the present method of directly correlating the treatment to the malady. Such an approach became possible only after the advances in pathological anatomy in the early nineteenth century had led to the recognition of local sites of disease in one organ or another, e.g., the heart, the kidneys, the liver. Humoral medicine, grounded as it was in a speculative theory, not in a detailed familiarity with the body, envisaged the person as sick in entirety, and so reached for an encompassing cure. However, the range of actual treatments was narrow: diet, perhaps fasting, purgatives, poultices, ointments, and frequently bleeding, carried out either by applying leeches or by opening a vein (Flaubert, *Madame Bovary,* [see "A Blood-Letting" in chapter 4]). Sometimes these measures served merely to weaken the patient further and to hasten death.

In this context it is hardly surprising that medical men enjoyed neither high prestige nor substantial income. Patients preferred first to resort to the herbal remedies traditional to folk and domestic medicine before seeking professional advice. Doctors spent much time traveling, mainly on horseback, to visit their patients at home. There they also had to deal with family members, who would be present at the consultation, and who, like the patients themselves, might hold strong opinions about the best course to follow. Since doctors possessed relatively little specialized knowledge, laypeople felt entitled to participate in treatment plans on an almost equal footing. The more affluent considered the doctor an employee not very much above the level of a servant. Medical attendants who gave unwelcome advice or who failed to show sufficient affability and deference were readily dismissed. On the other hand, those who found favor with their patients would over the years become confidential advisers and friends who could be entrusted with family problems

(Trollope, *Dr. Thorne* [see chapter 2]). In less positive relationships the doctors, for their part, would shield themselves by hiding obscurities and uncertainties behind quasi-scientific terminology. This led to another difficulty for patients: that of distinguishing reasonably competent physicians from the proliferation of quacks, mystics, magnetizers, and exorcisers who crowded the market with promises of magical cures that derived from secret nostrums and powers. Before mandatory control of the profession was enforced in Great Britain by the Medical Registration Act of 1858 and in the United States by laws such as that enacted in Illinois in 1877 authorizing state boards of examiners to accept diplomas only from reputable medical schools, the qualifications of those practicing medicine were open to extremely wide variations. As long as medicine itself was speculative, patients in turn had to engage in much speculation as to whose advice they should follow.

Cadavers and Instruments

Progress toward scientific medicine began with the practical exploration of anatomy through the dissection of cadavers in order to learn exactly how the body is made up and how its parts are connected to each other. Dissection of a cadaver remains to this day an essential facet of the medical school curriculum, the effective basis of all subsequent study. In this respect the twentieth-century convention reflects and replicates the learning process of medicine itself as a scientific discipline.

Despite some opposition from religious authorities on the grounds of desecration, the opening of the body for anatomical investigation and demonstration to students was initiated in the famous Italian medical schools at Bologna and Padua in the early fifteenth century. It was from Padua that Andreas Vesalius (1514–1564) graduated in 1537; for his finely illustrated *De Humani Corporis Fabrica* (1542; On the Structure of the Human Body) he is considered the founder of anatomy. His opus was important not only for the information it provided but also for its reliance on pragmatic observation in preference to abstract speculation. The move from dogmatism to empiricism was continued by the eighteenth-century Italian anatomist, Giovanni Morgagni (1682–1771) whose *De Sedibus et Causis Morborum per Anatomen Indagatis* (On the Sites and Causes of Diseases Investigated by Anatomy) appeared in 1761. Morgagni was the first to attempt to relate clinical symptoms with findings at autopsies. By posing the question "Ubi est morbus?" (Where is the disease?) he launched the idea that diseases are localized in one area of the body rather than the expression of a sweeping imbalance as humoral theories posited.

Vesalius and Morgagni paved the way for the fundamental discoveries of Marie-François-Xavier Bichat (1771–1801), the French pioneer of pathological anatomy whose research contributed greatly to making Paris the center of medical innovation in the earlier part of the nineteenth century. Bichat is reputed to have performed six hundred autopsies in one winter alone—dissection had to be seasonal because of the stench of putrefaction in the warmer months. The primary significance of Bichat's work lies in his recognition of distinctive lesions in particular organs as the signs of the disease that had caused sickness and death. In other words, he realized that the source of disease was a local abnormality. In his *General Anatomy Applied to Physiology and Medicine* (1801) he not only classified symptoms characteristic of disturbed organs but also identified the tissue of which organs are composed as the ultimate site of pathology. Through scrupulous analysis of what he saw in a long series of cadavers he was able to differentiate the types of disorder attacking pathologically deteriorated organs. Bichat's findings were of enormous importance in instigating one of the most momentous turning-points in medical history: the turn away from patient specificity to disease specificity in diagnosis and therapeutics (Eliot, *Middlemarch* [see "A Case of Typhoid Fever" in chapter 5]). Instead of regarding the entire body as in a state of imbalance, doctors in the wake of Bichat began aiming to pinpoint the singular lesion at the core of the patient's symptoms. That, of course, is the principle underlying modern medicine: to find by examination, and with the help of the battery of tests now at physicians' disposal, the location of the pathology where the symptoms originate in order then to apply therapeutic countermeasures. Bichat's recognition of the significance of lesions as the perceptible indication of disease ushers in a new era in the understanding of bodily disorders. A school for dissection opened in Paris in 1797 (Sue, *Les Mystères de Paris* [see chapter 3]), and by the mid to late 1830s physicians at London hospitals performed autopsies on almost two-thirds of their fatal cases.

The search for lesions in the living patient would not have been possible without the instrument devised less than two decades after Bichat's lifetime by his compatriot Laënnec. How Laënnec came up with the idea of the stethoscope is vividly described by Sherwin B. Nuland in *Doctors: The Biography of Medicine* (206–237). We take the stethoscope so much for granted as a portable diagnostic implement, indeed almost as the insignia of the medical profession, that it is difficult to imagine the extent to which it transformed practice. Before the stethoscope, doctors could try to deduce the patient's condition by putting an ear to the patient's chest or back in order to hear the sounds emitted by the heart and lungs.

This method, however, was not only primitive and unreliable, but it could also be offensive, especially to women patients who recoiled from a male physician's direct touch. An important advance was made by the Austrian Leopold Auenbrugger (1722–1809), who introduced percussion, which he described in his brief monograph *Inventum Novum* (1761; A New Invention). A skilled musician, Auenbrugger applied his knowledge of resonance, pitch, and tonal quality to the sounds emanating from patients' chests when they were tapped. He is reputed to have hit on this mode of examination from tapping his father's beer barrels and noticing that fluids and air spaces give out different sounds. Still, Laënnec's mediate or indirect auscultation made possible by the stethoscope was a great step forward from percussion because it afforded far more extensive and differentiated information. It was, too, more acceptable to patients by precluding the necessity for direct touch.

In its early version the stethoscope was rigid and applied to only one ear; later it was gradually modified to its present, familiar, dual-ear, flexible form. But even in its primitive shape it marks a major turning-point in the emergence of modern medicine through the emphasis initiated by Laënnec on the actual physical examination of patients. So long as doctors were dependent on their patients' subjective narratives of their symptoms and on surface observation, findings were bound to be primarily impressionistic. The stethoscope made possible the development toward a more objective diagnosis of disease by enabling doctors to draw distinctions between the sounds characteristic of specific disorders. Through expert, differentiating interpretation of the magnified sounds that can be heard through the stethoscope, doctors are able to ascertain what ails patients. But physical examination with this new instrument only attained its full value in combination with Bichat's discoveries at autopsies. The categoric ravages that Bichat saw in cadavers as the telltale signs of specific diseases could be directly related to the sounds emitted by the living person and picked up by means of the stethoscope. The connection between what was audible in the patient and what was visible in the cadaver enabled doctors to deduce a firmly grounded diagnostic taxonomy. Each disease—pleurisy, pneumonia, tuberculosis, inflammation of various areas of the heart—was found to have its characteristic sounds in living patients and to be confirmed by the damage revealed in cadavers. The conjunction of pathological anatomy with the stethoscope created a vital link between research and clinical practice and accomplished the transition from the speculative, theoretical mode of medicine typified by the belief in the humors to a scientific method rooted in pragmatically established facts.

Some fifty years after Bichat, studies in pathology again fostered a deeper and more refined grasp of disease processes (Eliot, *Middlemarch* [see "Lydgate's Ideals" in chapter 5]). In this instance the research was done in Germany, which took the lead in medical advances in the latter half of the nineteenth century. *Cellular Pathology*, published in 1858 by Rudolf Virchow (1821–1902), takes up where Bichat's premature death had forced him to leave off: in the comparative scrutiny of healthy and diseased tissues to see exactly in what ways they diverged from each other. Virchow was literally able to see more exactly than Bichat following the development of another essential instrument in the meanwhile: the decisive improvement in microscopes beginning in the 1830s and 1840s.

Magnifying lenses had been used certainly since at least the sixteenth century, but the spherical shape of the lenses and their tendency to disperse ordinary light into the various colors of the spectrum resulted in visual aberrations that severely reduced their efficacy as a scientific tool. The greater their magnifying power, the greater proportionately also was their liability to distortion. This optical obstacle was removed in 1829 by Joseph Jackson Lister (1786–1869) who devised the modern achromatic microscope,

With the adoption of this vastly more reliable instrument the gross pathology in which Bichat had engaged was replaced by microscopic pathology, which permitted far greater access to more minute elements of the body. The practical possibilities of the improved microscope were quickly harnessed; by 1843, for example, the microscopic department at Guy's Hospital in London was examining phlegm from lungs, blood, urine, and mother's milk, and two years later instruction in its use was incorporated into the medical school curriculum. Virchow, too, is reported constantly to have urged his students to learn to see microscopically. His own lasting distinction stems from his discovery that the real key to disease resides not so much in the disordered *structure* of the impaired cell but rather in its disordered *function*. So Bichat's pathologic anatomy was succeeded by Virchow's pathologic physiology, which focuses on the ways in which the sick cell acts. How it *looks* is only one pointer to the problem; how it *acts* is the crux of its defectiveness.

Shortly after Virchow, in the 1860s and 1870s the French Pierre-Charles-Alexandre Louis (1787–1872) initiated the numerical method which allowed for the quantification and graphic representation of temperature, pulse and respiration rates. Louis championed systematic analysis through statistics on the grounds that truth resides in objective facts.

Although improvement of the microscope preceded Virchow's research whereas the invention of the stethoscope followed Bichat's work, the two represent parallel instances of the fruitful interaction between new instruments and new conceptualizations of disease. After the stethoscope and the microscope, a long sequence of innovative instruments which allowed for viewing of internal organs was introduced into medical practice in the later nineteenth and the twentieth centuries. A urethracystic speculum became usable in 1827 after some twenty years of experimentation by a number of physicians. Similarly, the laryngoscope, also the product of lengthy trials, was brought to the United States at mid-century. The ophtahlmoscope was widely adopted only in the 1880s after some thirty years' work to simplify it. The endoscope proved a valuable diagnostic instrument from 1879 onward when a lens system with internal illumination was installed; rapid progress was then made in the inspection of the gullet, the stomach, the rectum, and the bladder, and the endoscope's potential was subsequently enlarged by the possibility of internal manipulation for the purposes of removing specimens and of therapeutic applications. A method for the direct insertion of a bronchoscope is attributed to the German laryngologist Gustav Killian in 1898. The first account of the use of a laparoscope for arthroscopy dates from 1921. Wilhelm Konrad Röntgen's x-rays (1895) mark another milestone in medicine's diagnostic repertoire, as does the introduction of the electrocardiograph at the dawn of the twentieth century. Much more recently various means of visualization have come into the forefront: both ultrasound and CAT (computer assisted tomography) scans were first described in articles published in 1939. Ultrasonic visualization of soft tissue was carried out in 1952, while tomography (computerized transverse axial scanning) in 1973 is credited to Godfrey Newbold Houndsfield, who was awarded the 1979 Nobel Prize in Medicine for this discovery. Nuclear magnetic resonance (MRI) to produce images of tissues was effected in 1973 by Paul Christian Lauterbur.

Germ Theory

Before medicine was put onto a scientific footing, the transmission of infectious diseases was also necessarily a matter of speculation. Devastating epidemics swept the world such as the Black Death in the fourteenth century, a form of the plague that decimated the population. So long as the ways in which these scourges originated and were disseminated remained unknown, there was no hope of curbing or preventing them. These ills, which spread like wildfire, were believed to spring from what was called "miasma," poisonous air thought to arise from swamps and marshy areas. Early in the nineteenth century, moralistic views were also prevalent: in the 1832 epidemic in the United States, cholera was regarded as a punishment of the thoughtless and immoral, unlikely to attack respectable people.

Even after microbes were discovered, they were not for some hundred and fifty years recognized as carriers of disease. The Dutch Antony Leeuwenhoek (1632–1723) was the first to see swarms of tiny moving mites through his rudimentary microscope. In 1677 he demonstrated to skeptical members of the Royal Society of London the validity of his discovery. Leeuwenhoek found microbes on all surfaces, including his own healthy teeth, and he also stumbled on the fact that they could be killed by heat, but he had no inkling of their potential noxiousness. Nor did the Italian naturalist Lazaro Spallanzani (1729–1799), although he made several salient observations about the animalcules, as they were named. He confirmed Leeuwenhoek's experience that heat killed them; on the other hand, he was surprised to see them surviving without air, sealed into a vacuum, and even more astonished at their capacity to multiply.

When the idea of contagion was first proposed, it met with such incredulity that its proponent was derided and ignored. In 1847 the Hungarian physician Ignaz Semmelweis (1818–1865), who was working in the huge hospital in Vienna, asserted that women died of childbed (puerperal) fever because they had been infected by putrid matter transmitted to them by their medical attendants. He based this revolutionary, dismaying contention on the astute observation that women who gave birth at home had a very low mortality, those who self-delivered even under the most adverse circumstances in alleyways and on streets had essentially no morbidity, whereas those hospitalized were felled at an alarming rate, regardless of the weather or the season. Watching hospital routine, Semmelweis saw doctors and medical students coming to assist women at childbirth straight from dissecting a putrid cadaver or lancing a pus-ridden boil or touching an infection-soaked sheet. He drew the conclusion that the physicians themselves were carrying the bacteria on their hands and transmitting them to their patients. He therefore instituted the measure of washing the hands in a chlorine solution until they were slippery and the cadaver smell had gone. The result was a dramatic decline in deaths from 18.3 percent to between 1.2 and 1.3 percent, an absolutely unprecedented drop. Nevertheless the majority of medical men continued to scoff at Semmelweis as a fanatic who was not of sound mind. He did suffer from a paranoid mental disorder in his final years, precipitated perhaps by the hounding he received. The negative reaction to his convincing argument is open to interpretation from a psychological angle as an expression of doctors' unwillingness to accept the responsibility (and the guilt) for the deaths they had unwittingly been causing.

Skepticism about the impact of animalcules in the spread of infections was widespread in the first half of the nineteenth century and dispelled only very slowly. The opposition that Lydgate encounters in the early 1830s in George Eliot's novel *Middlemarch* (see "The New Hospital" in chapter 5) to the establishment of an isolation hospital for fevers is wholly in keeping with the dominant opinion at that time. Even as late as 1861 there were virtually no public hospitals for infectious diseases in England. Many bizarre misconceptions flourished: for instance, lectures on clinical medicine given at the main hospital in Paris in 1834 cited nostalgia as one of the primary sources of typhoid fever. Although autopsies provided evidence of the damage wrought by various types of enteric fevers and so allowed for differential diagnosis, remarkably little was known about their causes or the paths of transmission. An important treatise was published in 1849 by the London physician Dr. John Snow, *On the Mode of Communication of Cholera*, proving that it was a water-borne infection.

The crucial impetus to an awareness of the destructive force of animalcules came, however, from a nonmedical scientist, the French Louis Pasteur (1822–1895), who was a chemist by profession. Pasteur, whose work is vividly evoked by Paul de Kruif in two chapters of *Microbe Hunters* (52–96, and 134–68), made his first great discovery at age twenty-six when he was consulted by a sugar beet distiller, some of whose vats were going bad instead of turning into alcohol, as they were supposed to do. The young chemist found that the difference between the good and the bad vats corresponded to the presence or absence of live yeasts to trigger the desired fermentation. In extending this line of research to rancid butter and putrefied meat, Pasteur came to realize the destructive power of microbes. He also proved by controlled experimentation what Leeuwenhoek and Spallanzani had seen microscopically: that the air is teeming with animalcules, and that they have the capacity to multiply. Pasteur thus drew on precise scientific methodologies to confirm what had previously been merely the outcome of good observation. The development of bacteriology was therefore important not just for the substance of its discoveries but also for its role as a vehicle to infuse the ideology of science into medical research. On the basis of his knowledge of the conditions under which bacteria thrive, Pasteur evolved the process still known as pasteurization, whereby harmful bacteria in, for example, milk, are killed by heating. The next problem he confronted was that of silkworms that were being ravaged by disease (this had serious economic implications since silkworms were essential to the French textile industry). After discerning globules in the sick worms under microscopic examination, Pasteur made a decisive breakthrough by identifying these parasites as not only the indicators of disease but as actually its cause. Coming from an entirely different sphere than Semmelweis, whose work remained largely unheeded, Pasteur reached the same conclusion: that germs were a deadly menace.

Pasteur is also central to the history of germ theory because he gave the lead in the production of a vaccine to protect creatures from the onslaught of animalcules. Pasteur worked initially with chickens in order to establish that inoculation with a weakened strain of the bacteria could create immunity. In May 1881 he gave a public demonstration of the effectiveness of this method by vaccinating sheep against the dreaded disease, anthrax. When the vaccinated cohort was unaffected by exposure to the infection while their unvaccinated counterparts succumbed, Pasteur was hailed as a savior throughout the world. His ultimate achievement was to apply the same principle to the invariably fatal effects of rabies. In 1885 he successfully tested the vaccine on a child that had been bitten by a mad dog. At last, near the close of the nineteenth century, scientific research brought not just an understanding of the transmission of infectious diseases but also a therapeutic antidote to save the lives of those attacked by lethal microbes. Nine years after Pasteur's rabies vaccine, in 1894, the French Emile Roux and the German Emil Behring made an antitoxin against diphtheria, an infection mainly of babies and children that choked them to death by blocking their air passages with pus. However, in remote locations this life-saving antitoxin was not readily available even some twenty years after its discovery. Martin Arrowsmith in Sinclair Lewis's novel has to travel a considerable distance to fetch it and arrives too late to save the child (see "A Case of Diphtheria" in chapter 7). In Mikhail Bulgakov's story, "The Steel Windpipe," set in a Russian hospital in 1916, the doctor has to resort to the old invasive method of a tracheotomy because he has none of the antitoxin (see chapter 8).

A German physician slightly junior to Pasteur, Robert Koch (1843–1910) made equally decisive discoveries in bacteriology in the later nineteenth century. Like Pasteur, Koch explored the resources of scientific research techniques for medicine. In contrast, however, to Semmelweis, who had based his detection of the cause of childbed fever simply on the observation of human behavior in the hospital, Koch, a brilliant microscopist, invoked the potential of science. By devising a system for staining microbes with a variety of colored dyes, he was able to see the differences between them. His insight that each disease is caused by a specific germ marks another major step in the battle against infectious diseases, for researchers learned to direct their efforts at particular targets. So Koch himself isolated the tuberculosis bacillus in 1882, and later that of Asiatic cholera, which invaded Europe in 1883.

Although Koch's tuberculin was not a cure for tuberculosis, as he had hoped, he was awarded the Nobel Prize for Medicine in 1905. A research institute was named after Koch in Germany in 1891, parallel to that established in France in 1888 named after Pasteur, prominent to this day. By the end of the nineteenth century, bacteriology had become an important facet of medical science (see Arrowsmith's fight against the plague [see "Plague" in chapter 7]). Still, public response to laboratory science remained mixed in the later nineteenth century, tending toward skepticism and even suspicion (Stevenson, *Dr. Jekyll and Mr. Hyde* [see chapter 6]). For while microscopy and analytical chemistry had relatively early diagnostic application in seriological tests, practical benefits to patients in the form of decisive interventions in the course of acute non-surgical diseases were for long scant.

Antisepsis, Asepsis, and Anesthesia

Germ theory was basic too in revolutionizing surgery in the second half of the nineteenth century. Up to then it had been a brutal business, consisting mainly of amputations, which were performed with the utmost speed while the patient was partially numbed by large amounts of liquor. Surgeons wore the same blood-sodden frock-coats year after year, and all the postoperative wounds in a ward were dressed with the same sponge from the same basin of water. Under these circumstances it is not surprising that the postoperative mortality rates ranged from 24 to 60 percent according to the hospital. Indeed, wound infection was considered an inevitable stage following surgery, for it was thought to be caused by the entry of oxygen into the tissue through the incision.

This prevailing belief in the concept of oxygen-induced putrefaction was contested by the British surgeon Joseph Lister (1827–1912), the son of the Lister who had devised the achromatic microscope. Lister was convinced that it was not the oxygen itself but something in the oxygen that triggered putrefaction once it entered the wound. Although Lister did not know of the work of Semmelweis, he thought along the same lines, namely that infection was imported into the patient from an identifiable external source. He read the articles Pasteur was then publishing about his experiments, which showed that putrefaction was caused in a previously sterilized solution of sugar through the introduction of microscopic organisms from the outside air. Applying this discovery to surgery, Lister concluded that contamination of the wound was brought on by invisible germ-laden particles entering from the surrounding air in the operating room.

Lister's next challenge was to find a means to kill the germs without injuring the patient's tissue. Carbolic acid had been successfully used in small quantities to combat the foul odors emanating from decomposed urban refuse, and by chance it was found to protect cattle grazing in neighboring fields from parasitic infections. Lister therefore chose to try a lint bandage dipped in carbolic acid on an open fracture of the leg; without a disinfectant such injuries frequently became infected so that the limb had to be amputated, and in almost half the cases death ensued from the resulting gangrene (Flaubert, *Madame Bovary* [see "Surgery" in chapter 4]). The fracture treated with the carbolic acid bandage healed within six weeks. After further successful experiments with the disinfectant on pus-filled abscesses, Lister published in 1867 a series of five papers in the *Lancet*, the leading British medical journal, under the title "The Antiseptic System: On a New Method of Treating Compound Fracture, Abscesses, etc.; with Observations on the Conditions of Suppuration." In a follow-up article in 1870 Lister gave the comparative mortality statistics: before antisepsis 16 deaths out of 35 cases, representing one in every two and a half; with antisepsis 6 deaths in 40 cases, representing one in every six and two-thirds.

Despite this strong evidence, Lister met with a certain amount of disbelieving opposition, more so in England than in other European countries. The grounds for British resistance are interesting: namely, the conviction that results from experiments in the laboratory are not transferrable to the phenomena of living tissue. This objection is a telling expression of the resistance among some doctors to converting medicine into a science. The principle of antisepsis found readier acceptance in countries such as France and Germany where the integration of science and medicine was already firmly established.

Antisepsis was superseded by the more radical asepsis before the end of the nineteenth century. Asepsis derives from the realization that organisms which may contaminate a wound are not solely air-borne; they reside too on the medical personnel's hands and instruments. While antisepsis aims to disinfect the wound, asepsis requires the rigorous sterilization of everything that will enter into the operative field. Asepsis is essentially a preventive approach designed to stop infection from ever contaminating the surgical wound. So the rituals now normative in surgery evolved: the scrubbing of hands, the boiling of instruments, the disinfectant cleansing of the patient's skin, the use of freshly laundered, germ-free gowns for the medical personnel and drapes for the patient. A number of technical innovations fostered asepsis. In 1883 the German surgeon Gustav Neuber designed a dust-free ventilating system for the private hospital he built; he was also the first to operate in a surgical cap and gown. In 1889 William Stewart Halsted of Baltimore popularized the use of rubber gloves. In 1886 another German surgeon, Ernst Bergmann, introduced sterilization by steam, and in 1891 he laid down the basic steps for achieving asepsis.

If antisepsis and asepsis made surgery much less risky, the discovery of general anesthesia fostered further great advances too. Not only was the patient liberated from the terrifying pain, but also extreme speed was no longer a necessity. Instead of being forcibly held down, as had been customary before anesthesia, the anesthetized patient lay in quiet repose so that the surgeon could take time to work carefully and more delicately. As general anesthesia became safer and safer, the length of operations could be extended, allowing surgeons to penetrate into deeper parts of the body. Without continuing improvements in anesthesia, today's dramatic surgeries, which often take many hours, would not have been feasible.

The invention of anesthesia was the first great contribution to medical science made by Americans. The discovery is enveloped in more contentiousness than any other in medical history, with at least three competitors claiming priority, all in the 1840s. The earliest of the three actually to use anesthesia was Crawford Williamson Long (1815–1878), a physician practicing in Georgia. In spring 1842 he removed a cyst from a patient who underwent the operation while breathing in ether through a towel soaked in the volatile liquid. In this method Long was importing into medicine the then current social habit of inhaling ether or nitrous oxide, popularly known as laughing gas. Ether induced a relaxed sleepiness, nitorus oxide a high hilarity. The effects of both were demonstrated as a form of entertainment by traveling "chemists" at theatrical shows in a circus-like atmosphere. Long may have derived his idea of exploiting the potential of ether for surgery from such a performance. But he did not publish his experiences until 1849 at the urging of friends. By then other claimants had come forward and were locked into legal disputes from which Long remained aloof.

One of the other contenders, Horace Wells (1815–1848), a dentist in Hartford, Connecticut, attended a laughing gas demonstration in December 1844, and began to extract teeth painlessly through use of the gas. Yet when he tried to prove the efficacy of his method to a critical medical audience in Boston in February 1845, the attempt was a dismal failure, probably because insufficient gas was administered. Wells was discredited; although he continued to experiment with ether and chloroform as well as nitrous oxide, and to pursue his claim, even going to Paris to petition the Academies of Science and of Medicine there, he was a broken man who committed suicide in 1848.

Meanwhile a successful demonstration of anesthesia by ether was given in Boston on 16 October 1846 by another dentist, William Thomas Green Morton (1819–1868). He had been in partnership with Wells in 1842–1843 before moving to Boston where he began to explore the possibilities of ether with the advice of the fourth person indirectly involved in the elaboration of anesthesia, the renowned Boston geologist and chemist Charles T. Jackson (1805–1880). Morton had a strong financial incentive to develop anesthesia for dentistry because he had devised a new type of plate to hold false teeth in place, but it only worked properly if old tooth roots and stumps were removed from patients' jaws—a painful procedure. Following an article in the *Boston Daily Journal* on 1 October 1846 describing Morton's extraction of an ulcerated tooth without pain while the patient was in an ether-induced sleep, he managed to have himself invited to demonstrate his technique at an operation on a tumor of the jaw at the Massachussetts General Hospital. Morton knew some of the staff at the hospital where he had taken courses. In November 1846 the *Boston Medical and Surgical Journal* published a positive article describing the twenty-five-minute operation, during which the patient remained free of pain. Although Morton is generally credited with the introduction of anesthesia, ironically Jackson too later entered the fray for the honor.

Following the introduction of anesthesia, the first appendectomy was performed in London in 1848. In the United States surgery grew and developed rapidly in response to the necessity of treating wounds in the Civil War. And Karl Landsteiner's discovery in 1900 of the specificty of blood types further expanded the possibilities of surgery by assuring the safety of transfusions.

Sociological Changes

The scientific and technological advances that took place in the course of the nineteenth century entailed sociological changes too. First and foremost, the status of the medical profession rose as physicians became more knowledgeable and therefore better able to help their patients. For instance, one outcome of the alliance between science and medicine was the synthesizing at an accelerated rate from the 1806s onward of effective drugs that provided immediate relief to the sick: barbituric acid, a sedative in 1863; digitalis, a heart regulator in 1869; salicylic acid (aspirin), an anti-inflammatory in 1874, and phenacetin, a pain-killer in 1887. As experts with the power to cure or at least to alleviate suffering, doctors began to command enormously increased prestige. So much so that medicine turned into a sacred profession set apart from others.

Another striking transformation occurred in the role of hospitals. Once the processes of transmitting infection were better understood and means to contain them incorporated into daily routine, hospitals could become places of healing rather than of death (Sue, *Les Mystères de Paris* [see chapter 3]). The incidence of the often lethal infections known in the mid-nineteenth century as "hospital fever" (cross-infection) and "wound fever" (gangrene) was significantly reduced as a result of the antiseptic and aseptic measures that became standard procedures. In the 1870s, twenty-four-hour staffing was introduced with trained nurses able to give skilled care.

In addition, the social stigma attached to hospitalization earlier in the century gradually disappeared. Because hospitals had grown out of almshouses and workhouses for the poor, they were literally the last resort of the indigent sick who had no homes or resources (Moore, *Esther Waters* [see chapter 10]). As medicine became more scientific, hospitals changed from being a refuge and receptacle for the socially disadvantaged to their current function as the site of the most avant-garde practice. Patients who were able to pay for medical attention began to patronize the specialized outpatient clinics that were set up in the 1880s for skin, ear, throat, eye, and chest diseases (Maugham, *Of Human Bondage*, [see "The Outpatient Clinic" in chapter 11]). But it continued to be the norm for the affluent classes to be tended at home even in serious illnesses. In mid-century, as Thomas Mann's *Buddenbrooks* shows, the family physician still habitually paid home visits, maintaining his traditional role of confidential friend from generation to generation, dispensing comfort while at the same time drawing on some innovations such as the stethoscope (Mann, *Buddenbrooks* [see chapter 9]). But later on the incremental complexity and, in many instances, size of the new instruments fostered a modification of attitudes toward hospitals. The early x-ray machines, for example, were so cumbersome that patients were obliged to go to where they were located instead of having the physician visit them at their homes. The number of hospitals in the United States rose from 178 in 1872 to more than 4000 by 1910. Separate pavilions were constructed with improved ventilation as part of the efforts to minimize cross-infections. These new structures also served to segregate charity from paying patients who were cossetted in luxurious hotel-like settings where their meals were served on linens, china, and silver so as to replicate the lifestyle to which they were accustomed. From the physicians' point of view, hospitalization had therapeutic benefits: it allowed for closer supervision of patients and their removal from the possible tensions of home surroundings. Incidentally, it also augmented doctors' power (and income by reducing the time they spent in travel). On the other hand, the removal of patients from their homes and the reduction of the actual time doctor and patient spent together altered their relationship by fostering a greater emotional distance and impersonality. The scientific focus on localized disease reduced the attention paid to the patient's social context and personality.

Hospitals also came to assume much greater importance in medical training. As medicine switched from a speculative to a scientific model, medical education had to become far more rigorous. In the United States, President Charles Eliot of Harvard University instituted a thorough reform of the medical curriculum in 1871. The previous two-year program consisting largely of theoretical, didactic lectures in random sequence was expanded into a three-year course in which anatomy, physiology, and chemistry came to play an ever more central part. The experimental sciences gained unprecedented prominence with hands-on laboratory experience mandated for every student. This concentration on the practical aspects continued in bedside learning, which was increasingly assimilated into medical training over the nineteenth century. Although in the late eighteenth century already students were urged to gain familiarity with disease by "walking the wards," as it was called, this remained a voluntary, informal facet of medical education in which students were merely passive spectators and listeners. But when speculative "library" medicine was superseded by scientific methodologies, more emphasis was put onto experiential learning. By the end of the nineteenth century, as Maugham's *Of Human Bondage* (see chapter 11) illustrates, medical students were active participants in clinical care, learning to use diagnostic instruments as well as to decide on the best therapeutics. In the hospital's new teaching capacity the outpatient clinics assumed a vital role in screening, selecting, and procuring patients. By a process of triage from a large pool of prospective patients, those with interesting diseases were admitted to the hospital. This system could be of mutual benefit as the sickest were given special attention while physicians acquired the patients they needed for teaching purposes.

The appearance of women doctors in the latter third of the nine-teenth century marks a further significant sociological change. Their hard struggle to gain admission and acceptance in the profession in the United States and Great Britain is briefly reviewed in the prefatory remarks to Sarah Orne Jewett's *A Country Doctor* (see chapter 12) and to Arthur Conan Doyle's "The Doctors of Hoyland" (see chapter 13). Women physicians are the subject of a number of American and British fictions published between the late 1870s and the mid-1890s. They reflect the ability of these "new women" to function as professionals and the effect of their relatively liberated status on their personal lives. However, the percentage of women students in American medical schools dropped precipitously from a high of 18.2 percent in 1893–1894 to a low of 4.6 percent in 1944. This sharp decline was a direct consequence of the absorption of women's medical colleges into coeducational schools be-tween 1884 and 1903; women were supposed to be admitted to the newly consolidated institutions, but in fact this agreement was not hon-ored. Only after World War II did the numbers of women doctors gradu-ally rise again.

Apart from its wider interest as an aspect of women's fight for emancipation from the strict patriarchal limitations still imposed on them in the later nineteenth century, their participation in medicine had im-mediate repercussions within the medical world in the ongoing debate about the nature and purpose of medicine. The controversy testifies to a continuing resistance to science by some members of the profession. At the commencement address in Cincinnati in 1877, for example, Dr. Nathanael West maintained that "The dignity and sanctity of the medical profession, its chief excellence is, not that it is scientific, but that it is redemptive." Exactly what was meant by "redemptive" is hard to fathom; in its religious undertones it harks back to the older vision of the phy-sician as a "missionary to the bedside." Women in particular debated whether their style of medicine should differ from men's in being "ma-ternal," as Elizabeth Blackwell (1821–1910), the first woman doctor suggested, or whether they too should embrace the scientific approach, as others such as Mary Putnam Jacobi (1842–1906) argued.

This debate in turn opens up onto the even deeper issue of the doctor-patient relationship: in what ways and to what extent was it modified by scientific advances? It was bound to be affected by the vast expansion of physicians' expertise and their consequent capacity to offer their patients more efficacious treatments. The growth in doctors' com-mand of scientific knowledge inevitably led to a cumulative disparity between them and their patients with whom they no longer necessarily shared common assumptions—let alone, knowledge—about the origins of diseases and their optimal treatment, as they had done in the days of humoral medicine. The gulf widened as doctors became less dependent on patients' subjective accounts for information about their condition, and turned increasingly to objective measurements derived extraneously from scientific modes of examination.

Taken to extremes, these developments resulted in the later twentieth century in the tensions that beset the doctor-patient relationship, and at worst may become manifest in reciprocal distrust, and at times litigation. These tendencies did not yet amount to a serious threat in the later nineteenth century for a variety of reasons. Technology had not yet attained the supremacy it achieved in the course of the twentieth century through additional sophisticated instrumentation, the refinement of biochemistry, not to mention molecular biology and genetic engineering. Economic factors proved a determinant too, especially in the United States where the overproduction of doctors in the closing two decades of the nineteenth century following the tripling in the number of medical schools from 52 in 1850 to 160 in 1900 posed a serious challenge to physicians through the amount of competition they faced. Daniel W. Cathell's *Book on the Physician Himself* is a reflection of this situation as he spells out the conduct required to achieve "reputation and success" (see chapter 14). By this euphemistic phrase he clearly means how to attract and keep patients, and so assure financial security. While Cathell advocates the judicious use of scientific instruments (not least to impress patients), he also insists repeatedly on the worth of such social factors as good manners, a clean appearance, and geniality.

The foundations for modern medicine were laid in the course of the nineteenth century through momentous advances in the *basic sciences* that produced a much more accurate understanding of disease processes than had previously been attainable. Improved instrumentation such as the achromatic microscope and huge leaps in laboratory techniques opened up radically new insights into the causes and modes of transmission of many diseases. But for most of the century the gap between medical knowledge and therapeutic activity only widened. The brisk progress in microscopic pathology and biological chemistry served merely to highlight the relative stagnation in therapeutics. In contrast to the usefulness of microscopy and analytical chemistry in diagnostics, the immediate therapeutic spin-offs of laboratory science for patients were fairly small until the very end of the century. Discontent with science is aptly summarized in the German slogan demanding cures not classifications. Only in the twentieth century were patients able to reap the benefits from the advances in the basic sciences made in the nineteenth century, as the experiments performed in the laboratory bore fruit in a spate of medications and procedures that eventually evolved from the new understandings gradually achieved on ground that had been explored and mapped in the latter part of the previous century.

The medical episodes in nineteenth-century literary works flesh out history in significant ways by revealing the extremely erratic pace of progress, the intensity of opposition in some quarters, and the combination of often irrational factors obstructing any innovation. It is tempting to envisage the advance of medicine as a triumphal conquest of disease held back only temporarily by occasional setbacks. The actual circumstances were far more complex, largely because doctors had to exercise their calling in a social reality that was generally conservative, at best suspicious of innovations, and at times downright hostile. Doctors had to make medical judgments on limited information, accommodate all sorts of prejudices, address individual needs and lifestyles, deal with patients at all social levels with vastly differing expectations, work within existing institutions while also trying to reform them, and adjudicate the scientific, ethical, financial, and status considerations attendant on their role, which was itself changing. The literary excerpts in this anthology reflect this quite complicated, even contradictory situation by showing the various impediments to progress that resulted in shortfall. For example, Lydgate in George Eliot's *Middlemarch* is very well trained and informed of the latest findings, yet is thwarted from applying them by the townspeople's resistance to any departure from their established customs. On the other hand, Sinclair Lewis's Martin Arrowsmith makes the deliberate choice to ruin his controlled experiment with the bacteriophage by vaccinating everyone at the height of a deadly epidemic of the plague; his humanitarian commitment as a doctor to alleviate suffering and save lives overrides his obligation as a research scientist. On a less idealistic level, Daniel W. Cathell in his *Book on the Physican Himself*, by categorically warning young practitioners against an excess of science, is bowing to the social reality that patients will more likely flock to a likable doctor than to one who tries to dazzle them with fancy scientific concepts and frightening instruments.

The literary texts thus serve to modify the tendency to view medical progress in the nineteenth century in a simplistic manner. Compromises have constantly to be negotiated; concessions are demanded of both doctors and patients that neither group is prepared to make. The implementation of medical progress in the social reality of the time was no easy matter.

1

An Introduction to the Ethical Basis of Medical Practice

The Hippocratic Oath and Its Successors

The swearing of the Hippocratic Oath at graduation represents physicians' rite of passage into a profession with special prerogatives and obligations. The oath is a covenant, a pledge of trust dedicating physicians to their chosen task of curing or alleviating suffering, or at the very least doing no harm. Although it has over the centuries been reformulated or expanded, it continues to form the ethical basis of medical practice.

Hippocrates was born on the Greek island of Kos about 460 B.C., the son of the healer, Heraclides. There is little reliable information concerning his life. He is known to have practiced empirical medicine, i.e., devolving from observation of and comparison with previous cases. Such an experiential method was the optimal mode before the advent of the experimental sciences in the nineteenth century.

The Hippocratic Oath opens with invocation of Greek divinities: according to mythology, Apollo was the god endowed with powers of healing which were gradually transferred to a lesser deity, Aesculapius and his legendary daughters, Hygiea and Panacea. This classical version of the oath has sometimes been deemed pagan; an alternative opening suitable for Christians dates from the tenth or eleventh century: "Blessed be God the Father of our Lord Jesus Christ, who is blessed for ever and ever" (see "The Christian Hippocratic Oath"). Whatever its exact wording (and there are many variants), the oath is short and incisive in its

23

substance. First and foremost it declares a dual commitment: to the traditions of medicine as they have been taught and as they are to be transmitted to future generations; and to the well-being of patients to the best of the physician's ability and judgment. But also conspicuous in the oath are the prohibitions it imposes: to desist from giving deadly medications on request, from providing an abortifacient, from cutting persons suffering from stones (because this should be done only by specialized experts), and from taking advantage of access to homes by instigating mischief or indulging in seduction. It is remarkable that the Hippocratic Oath, taken as a whole, devotes a larger proportion of its imperatives to forbidding certain types of negative behavior than to defining the positives.

Before the legal regulation of physicians, which was slow and erratic, the Oath was not consistently administered. Laws to limit the practice of medicine to instructed persons were enacted in European states in 1224, 1347, and 1365. In England Henry VIII granted a charter to the Barber-Surgeons Guild in 1512 and to the Royal College of Physicians in 1518. These ordinances conferred on the members of these associations the right of training and examining newcomers to the profession, and like the Hippocratic Oath mandated scrupulously moral relations with patients as well as enumerating members' obligations to each other. The British Medical Registration Act of 1858 marks a major milestone in requiring all aspirants to the profession to have their qualifications approved before they could be registered to practice. In the United States licensing and proper professional regulation were introduced in the 1870s and 1880s. The stiffened enforcement of requirements is typified by the 1877 law in Illinois that empowered a state board of examiners to accept diplomas only from reputable schools.

The clarification of standards was significantly furthered by the publication in 1803 of *Medical Ethics; or, a Code of Institutes and Precepts, Adapted to the Professional Conduct of Physicians and Surgeons* (reprinted in *Percival's Medical Ethics*. Ed. Chauncey D. Leake. Baltimore: Williams & Wilkins, 1927, 65–166). It was written by a British physician, Thomas Percival (1740–1804) at the request of the trustees of the Manchester Infirmary to settle a dispute among its staff. Running to over one hundred pages, this document discusses professional conduct under four headings: "Relative to Hospitals or Other Medical Charities," "In Private or General Practice," "Towards Apothecaries," and "In Certain Cases Which Require a Knowledge of Law." The most extensive section is that devoted to private or general practice. It sets out a combination of moral and practical guidelines, advocating strict observance of secrecy and delicacy, temperance, punctuality, avoidance of interference, respect for seniority, consultations in difficult cases, continued attendance on incurables, discouragement of quacks and nostrums, and the appropriate ways to collect fees.

The *Code of Ethics* adopted by the newly founded American Medical Association in 1847 deals with many of the same topics Percival addressed, at times in wording that echoes his verbatim. "Ethics" means conduct in the widest sense, covering in its three chapters first "The Duties of Physicians to the Patients and the Obligations of Patients to their Physicians" (No. 2), secondly the duties of physicians to each other and to the profession at large, and thirdly the duties of the profession to the public and the obligations of the public to the profession. Since this *Code of Ethics* supplements but does not replace the Hippocratic Oath, there is here no insistence on negative prohibitions. The entire document concentrates on what is desirable in the interaction between physician and patient. General principles are laid down in the first two articles on the duties of physicians to their patients. The key phrase in the very opening sentence is that the physician's mind ought "to be imbued with the greatness of his mission." This articulates the ideal image of the physician at that time as a missionary to the bedside, or, as the *Code* puts it in similarly religious terms, "the minister of hope and comfort to the sick." Other major injunctions include the strict observation of "secrecy and delicacy," the uniting of "tenderness with firmness, and condescension with authority," and the exercise in every case of "attention, steadiness, and humanity." Articles three through seven concern specifics in the conduct of medical practice: the frequency of visits, the necessity of steering a wary course between gloom and "timely notice of danger" to patients' friends and possibly even to patients themselves, the obligation not to abandon incurables, the recourse to consultations, and finally, the opportunity that physicians have for health education. Some of these articles are obviously restatements of traditional lore ("secrecy and delicacy," incurables, consultations), but others are innovative, particularly the problem of truth-telling and the recognition that physicians can influence their patients to amend their health habits. The 1847 *Code* thus ranges from the quasi-religious foundations of medical practice to social issues that have come to assume increasing importance in the past hundred and fifty years.

Another novel and unique departure, never replicated in later similar statements of principles, is the inclusion of the "Obligations of Patients to their Physicians." The tone of this section is quite defensive. The doctors straightaway proclaim themselves as performing "so many important and arduous duties towards the community, and as required to make so many sacrifices of comfort, ease, and health for the welfare of those who avail themselves of their services" that, they argue, they "have a right to expect and require, that their patients should entertain a just sense of the duties they owe to their medical attendants." This declaration, tactful and cautiously phrased though it is, introduces into the relationship between doctor and patient the principle of reciprocity absent in the Hippocratic Oath and in Percival's *Medical Ethics*. Some of the following nine articles deal with purely practical arrangements such as sending for the doctor in the morning if possible, not delaying consultations until the disease has advanced to a violent stage, and giving reasons for dismissal. Others devolve from conditions at that period, such as the injunction to select as medical adviser "one who has received a regular medical education." Similarly, the argument for confiding the care of the family to one physician on a long-term basis stems from the mid-nineteenth-century belief in the patient-specificity of treatment: "for a medical man who has become acquainted with the peculiarities of constitution, habits, and predispositions, of those he attends, is more likely to be successful in his treatment, than one who does not possess that knowledge." Yet often patients are firmly placed in a subordinate position, enjoined to communicate "faithfully and unreservedly," to answer questions briskly, to obey the physician's prescriptions promptly and implicitly, and not to consult several physicians simultaneously. Lastly, patients are reminded that the worth of a physician's services are beyond monetary payment. This section of the 1847 *Code* reveals the medical profession's relative insecurity before its authority became grounded in science.

In contrast to the five thousand and six hundred words of the 1847 *Code of Ethics*, the 1980 American Medical Association's *Principles of Medical Ethics* runs to just two hundred and fifty words. The very terseness of the wording emphasizes the binding nature of the principles enunciated. The eight articles spell out directly and cogently the major imperatives: "compassion and respect for human dignity" comes first, and honesty second; safeguarding patients' confidentiality is also a high priority. These are by and large reiterations of the ethos underlying the Hippocratic Oath. So the Oath's obligation to teach is reformulated into the commitment "to continue to study, apply and advance scientific knowledge, make relevant information available to patients, colleagues, and the public." Two new provisions are included: one (article 6) asserts the right to freedom of choice: "to choose whom to serve, with whom to associate and the environment in which to provide medical services" (except in emergencies). The other concerns the commitment to participate in activites contributing to an improved community, and, while respecting the law, to seek changes in requirements contrary to patients' best interests. The 1980 *Principles of Medical Ethics* recognize physicians' obligation to society as a whole as well as to individual patients. Physicians' privileges are widened in the claim to freedom of choice but so are their responsibilities.

The Hippocratic Oath has in recent years been experimentally revised in some medical schools. In 1986, for instance, graduates of Tufts Medical School chose to underscore the importance of preventive medicine by including this phrase: "I will prevent disease whenever I can, for prevention is better than cure." This clause amplifies, in twentieth-century terms, the injunction in the 1847 *Code* to promote and strengthen patients' good resolutions. As the value of preventive medicine (e.g., regular exercise, sensible nutrition, not smoking, control of blood pressure) has come to be better understood, the physician's educational function has moved into the foreground. The Tufts graduates also vowed "to remember that there is an art in medicine as well as science, and that warmth, sympathy, and understanding may outweigh the surgeon's knife or the chemist's drug." This reminder of the need for a humane approach reiterates the 1847 *Code*'s notion of "tenderness," allied now to the recognition that medicine as science has to be tempered by medicine as an art.

In all the various codes of conduct, the ethical guidelines are largely general. So the Hippocratic Oath prohibits "intentional ill-doing," while its 1980 successor prescribes "honorable behavior." The sole exception is the Hippocratic Oath's ban on abortion. Apart from this, the ethical dilemmas that preoccupy us today, notably end-of-life questions such as euthanasia or assisted suicide or the right to withhold life support, are wholly absent. These issues were not part of nineteenth-century medical practice because expectations were quite different. The average life-span was far shorter, conditions were harsher, especially for the poor, so that suffering and early death were accepted as the norm. Tuberculosis was a common scourge, and epidemics of diphtheria and scarlet fever contributed to a high infant and child mortality. Many current dilemmas have arisen as a direct result of twentieth-century technology: respirators, dialysis, and artificial feeding tubes permit the continuation of life beyond what would have been the natural point of death a century ago; at the same time they create the ethical problems of choice we face today. Another cogent example is the use of ultrasound and amniocentesis for the intrauterine diagnosis of defects in the fetus so that parents must make agonizing decisions about whether or not to terminate the pregnancy.

By contrast, ethics in the nineteenth century centered on the doctor-patient relationship, that is, the appropriate standards of reciprocal behavior. The collection of fees frequently proved a thorny matter. Physicians were regarded as employees who could be readily dismissed if they seemed unsatisfactory. Such temperamental behavior on patients' part (see Trollope, *Dr. Thorne*, ["Lady Arabella" and "Sir Roger" in chapter 2] prompted an insistence on doctors' part on the maintenance of their dignity as professionals. For instance, if they were offered refreshments, as was the custom, especially in the country, they did not want to take them with the servants. This clearly reveals the extent to which doctors had to assert themselves in order to achieve a certain measure of respect and social status. A more serious and lasting quandary was whether it was advisable to tell dying or mortally sick patients the truth about their condition and prognosis. The 1847 *Code* comes out in favor of gently imparting the truth, but opinion remained divided on the grounds that bad news might undermine and discourage patients psychologically and so lessen their prospects of recovery (see Mann, *Buddenbrooks* ["Pneumonia" in chapter 9]).

Consideration of the successive codes of conduct for physicians shows both the basic constants underlying proper professional behavior and the modifications in the wake of medical progress and the changing status of physicians. From the first delineation of the conventions governing physicians' transactions with their patients in the Hippocratic Oath, the highest moral expectations are laid down and reiterated in each restatement of the principles. Integrity and discretion are the immutable fundamentals. By the mid-nineteenth century the need for reciprocal respect was spelled out as medical men became more assured of their status with advances in their knowledge. The concept of social activism was added quite recently in recognition of the importance of preventive medicine and of the necessity for direct input into social reality.

The amendments introduced since the Hippocratic Oath raise several questions. Have the ethical issues become more complicated as a result of scientific and technological advances? Does the capacity to prolong life (in some instances) also entail decisions about the quality of life? Who has the ultimate right to make such decisions: patient, or doctor, or jointly? What about the costs? Should the teaching of ethics be a part of every medical school curriculum? Is medicine's growing power to control life and death as much a burden as an asset?

The Hippocratic Oath

Oath of Hippocrates of Kos, Fifth Century B.C.

I swear by Apollo the physician, by Aesculapius, Hygeia, and Panacea, and I take to witness all the gods, all the goddesses, to keep according to my ability and my judgment the following oath:

To consider dear to me as my parents him who taught me this art; to live in common with him and if necessary to share my goods with him; to look upon his children as my own brothers, to teach them this art if they so desire without fee or written promise; to impart to my sons and the sons of the master who taught me and to the disciples who have enrolled themselves and have agreed to the rules of the profession, but to these alone, the precepts and the instruction. I will prescribe a regimen for the good of my patients according to my ability and my judgment and never do harm to anyone. To please no one will I prescribe a deadly drug, nor give advice which may cause his death. Nor will I give a woman a pessary to procure abortion. But I will preserve the purity of my life and my art. I will not cut for stone, even for patients in whom the disease is manifest; I will leave this operation to be performed by specialists in this art. In every house where I come I will enter only for the good of my patients, keeping myself far from all intentional ill-doing and all seduction, and especially from the pleasures of love with women or with men, be they free or slaves. All that may come to my knowledge in the exercise of my profession or outside of my profession or in daily commerce with men, which ought not to be spread abroad, I will keep secret and will never reveal. If I keep this oath faithfully, may I enjoy my life and practice my art, respected by all men and in all times; but if I swerve from it or violate it, may the reverse be my lot.

The Christian Hippocratic Oath

From the Oath According to Hippocrates
Insofar As a Christian May Swear It

Blessed be God the Father of our Lord Jesus Christ, who is blessed for ever and ever; I lie not.

I will bring no stain upon the learning of the medical art. Neither will I give poison to anybody though asked to do so, nor will I suggest such a plan. Similarly I will not give treatment to women to cause abortion, treatment neither from above nor from below. But I will teach this art, to those who require to learn it, without grudging and without an indenture. I will use treatment to help the sick according to my ability and judgment. And in purity and in holiness I will guard my art. Into whatsoever houses I enter, I will do so to help the sick, keeping myself free from all wrongdoing, intentional or unintentional, tending to death or to injury, and from fornication with bond or free, man or woman. Whatsoever in the course of practice I see or hear (or outside my practice in social intercourse) that ought not to be published abroad, I will not divulge, but consider such things to be holy secrets. Now if I keep this oath and break it not, may God be my helper in my life and art, and may I be honoured among all men for all time. If I keep faith, well; but if I forswear myself may the opposite befall me.

31

American Medical Association's 1847 Code of Ethics

Of the Duties of Physicians to Their Patients and of the Obligations of Patients to Their Physicians

Duties of Physicians to Their Patients

1. A physician should not only be ever ready to obey the calls of the sick, but his mind ought also to be imbued with the greatness of his mission, and the responsibility he habitually incurs in its discharge. Those obligations are the more deep and enduring, because there is no tribunal other than his own conscience to adjudge penalties for carelessness or neglect. Physicians should, therefore, minister to the sick with due impressions of the importance of their office; reflecting that the ease, the health, and the lives of those committed to their charge, depend on their skill, attention and fidelity. They should study, also, in their department, so to unite tenderness with firmness, and condescension with authority, as to inspire the minds of their patients with gratitude, respect and confidence.

2. Every case committed to the charge of a physician should be treated with attention, steadiness, and humanity. Reasonable indulgence should be granted to the mental imbecility and caprices of the sick.

From *Percival's Medical Ethics*, Chauncey D. Leake, ed. (Baltimore: Williams & Wilkins, 1927), pp. 219–225.

Secrecy and delicacy, when required by peculiar circumstances, should be strictly observed; and the familiar and confidential intercourse to which physicians are admitted in their professional visits, should be used with discretion, and with the most scrupulous regard to fidelity and honor. The obligation of secrecy extends beyond the period of professional services;—none of the privacies of personal and domestic life, no infirmity of disposition or flaw of character observed during professional attendance, should ever be divulged by him except when he is imperatively required to do so. The force and necessity of this obligation are indeed so great, that professional men have, under certain circumstances, been protected in their observance of secrecy by courts of justice.

3. Frequent visits to the sick are in general requisite, since they enable the physician to arrive at a more perfect knowledge of the disease, to meet promptly every change which may occur, and also tend to preserve the confidence of the patient. But unnecessary visits are to be avoided, as they give useless anxiety to the patient, tend to diminish the authority of the physician, and render him liable to be suspected of interested motives.

4. A physician should not be forward to make gloomy prognostications, because they savor of empiricism, by magnifying the importance of his services in the treatment or cure of the disease. But he should not fail, on proper occasions, to give to the friends of the patient timely notice of danger when it really occurs; and even to the patient himself, if absolutely necessary. This office, however, is so peculiarly alarming when executed by him, that it ought to be declined whenever it can be assigned to any other person of sufficient judgment and delicacy. For, the physician should be the minister of hope and comfort to the sick; that, by such cordials to the drooping spirit, he may smooth the bed of death, revive expiring life, and counteract the depressing influence of those maladies which often disturb the tranquillity of the most resigned in their last moments. The life of a sick person can be shortened not only by the acts, but also by the words or the manner of a physician. It is, therefore, a sacred duty to guard himself carefully in this respect, and to avoid all things which have a tendency to discourage the patient and to depress his spirits.

5. A physician ought not to abandon a patient because the case is deemed incurable; for his attendance may continue to be highly useful to the patient, and comforting to the relatives around him, even in the last period of a fatal malady, by alleviating pain and other symptoms, and by soothing mental anguish. To decline attendance, under such circumstances, would be sacrificing to fanciful delicacy, and mistaken liberality,

that moral duty, which is independent of, and far superior to, all pecuniary consideration.

6. Consultations should be promoted in difficult or protracted cases, as they give rise to confidence, energy, and more enlarged views in practice.

7. The opportunity which a physician not unfrequently enjoys of promoting and strengthening the good resolutions of his patients, suffering under the consequences of vicious conduct, ought never to be neglected. His counsels, or even remonstrances, will give satisfaction, not offence, if they be proffered with politeness, and evince a genuine love of virtue, accompanied by a sincere interest in the welfare of the person to whom they are addressed.

Obligations of Patients to Their Physicians

1. The members of the medical profession, upon whom is enjoined the performance of so many important and arduous duties towards the community, and who are required to make so many sacrifices of comfort, ease, and health, for the welfare of those who avail themselves of their services, certainly have a right to expect and require, that their patients should entertain a just sense of the duties which they owe to their medical attendants.

2. The first duty of a patient is, to select as his medical adviser one who has received a regular professional education. In no trade or occupation, do mankind rely on the skill of an untaught artist; and in medicine, confessedly the most difficult and intricate of the sciences, the world ought not to suppose that knowledge is intuitive.

3. Patients should prefer a physician whose habits of life are regular, and who is not devoted to company, pleasure, or to any pursuit incompatible with his professional obligations. A patient should, also, confide the care of himself and family, as much as possible, to one physician, for a medical man who has become acquainted with the peculiarities of constitution, habits, and predispositions, of those he attends, is more likely to be successful in his treatment, than one who does not possess that knowledge.

A patient who has thus selected his physician, should always apply for advice in what may appear to him trivial cases, for the most fatal results often supervene on the slightest accidents. It is of still more importance that he should apply for assistance in the forming stage of violent diseases; it is to a neglect of this precept that medicine owes much of the uncertainty and imperfection with which it has been reproached.

4. Patients should faithfully and unreservedly communicate to their physician the supposed cause of their disease. This is the more important, as many diseases of a mental origin simulate those depending on external causes, and yet are only to be cured by ministering to the mind diseased. A patient should never be afraid of thus making his physician his friend and adviser; he should always bear in mind that a medical man is under the strongest obligations of secrecy. Even the female sex should never allow feelings of shame or delicacy to prevent their disclosing the seat, symptoms, and causes of complaints peculiar to them. However commendable a modest reserve may be in the common occurrences of life, its strict observance in medicine is often attended with the most serious consequences, and a patient may sink under a painful and loathsome disease, which might have been readily prevented had timely intimation been given to the physician.

5. A patient should never weary his physician with a tedious detail of events or matters not appertaining to his disease. Even as relates to his actual symptoms, he will convey much more real information by giving clear answers to interrogatories, than by the most minute account of his own framing. Neither should he obtrude upon his physician the details of his business nor the history of his family concerns.

6. The obedience of a patient to the prescriptions of his physician should be prompt and implicit. He should never permit his own crude opinions as to their fitness, to influence his attention to them. A failure in one particular may render an otherwise judicious treatment dangerous, and even fatal. This remark is equally applicable to diet, drink, and exercise. As patients become convalescent, they are very apt to suppose that the rule prescribed for them may be disregarded, and the consequence, but too often, is a relapse. Patients should never allow themselves to be persuaded to take any medicine whatever, that may be recommended to them by the self-constituted doctors and doctresses, who are so frequently met with, and who pretend to possess infallible remedies for the cure of every disease. However simple some of their prescriptions may appear to be, it often happens that they are productive of much mischief, and in all cases they are injurious, by contravening the plan of treatment adopted by the physician.

7. A patient should, if possible, avoid even the friendly visits of a physician who is not attending him—and when he does receive them, he should never converse on the subject of his disease, as an observation may be made, without any intention of interference, which may destroy his confidence in the course he is pursuing, and induce him to neglect the directions prescribed to him. A patient should never send for a

consulting physician without the express consent of his medical attendant. It is of great importance that physicians should act in concert; for
although their modes of treatment may be attended with equal success
when employed singly, yet conjointly they are very likely to be productive of disastrous results.

8. When a patient wishes to dismiss his physician, justice and common courtesy require that he should declare his reasons for so doing.

9. Patients should always, when practicable, send for their physician
in the morning, before his usual hour of going out; for, by being early
aware of the visits he has to pay during the day, the physician is able to
apportion his time in such a manner as to prevent an interference of
engagements. Patients should also avoid calling on their medical adviser
unnecessarily during the hours devoted to meals or sleep. They should
always be in readiness to receive the visits of their physician, as the
detention of a few minutes is often of serious inconvenience to him.

10. A patient should, after his recovery, entertain a just and enduring
sense of the value of the services rendered him by his physician; for these
are of such a character, that no mere pecuniary acknowledgement can
repay or cancel them.

American Medical Association's 1980
Principles of Medical Ethics

The medical profession has long subscribed to a body of ethical statements developed primarily for the benefit of the patient. As a member of this profession, a physician must recognize responsibility not only to patients, but also to society, to other health professionals, and to self. The following Principles adopted by the American Medical Association are not laws, but standards of conduct which define the essentials of honorable behavior for the physician.

I. A physician shall be dedicated to providing competent medical service with compassion and respect for human dignity.

II. A physician shall deal honestly with patients and colleagues, and strive to expose those physicians deficient in character or competence, or who engage in fraud or deception.

III. A physician shall respect the law and also recognize a responsibility to seek changes in those requirements which are contrary to the best interests of the patient.

IV. A physician shall respect the rights of patients, of colleagues, and of other health professionals, and shall safeguard patient confidences within the constraints of the law.

V. A physician shall continue to study, apply and advance scientific knowledge, make relevant information available to patients, colleagues, and the public, obtain consultation, and use the talents of other health professionals when indicated.

VI. A physician shall, in the provision of appropriate patient care, except in emergencies, be free to choose whom to serve, with whom to associate, and the environment in which to provide medical services.

VII. A physician shall recognize a responsibility to participate in activities contributing to an improved community.

2

An Old Style Doctor

An Introduction to Selections from Anthony Trollope's Dr. Thorne

Anthony Trollope (1815–1892) was a prolific writer who published over forty novels and many short stories. His output is the more remarkable in light of the fact that he also had a distinguished full-time career in the British postal service where his achievements include the organization of mail in Ireland and to Egypt. As a novelist he enjoyed considerable acclaim during his lifetime, and there has recently been a major revival of interest with the re-issue of all his novels in paperback.

Dr. Thorne (1858) is a relatively early work, the second in the series known as the "Barsetshire" novels because they all take place in this particular county not too far from London. The first and most famous of the sequence, *Barchester Towers* (1857) deals with the political jostling for rank and power among the clergymen at the town's cathedral. The Barsetshire cycle, comprising five novels published in the decade between 1857 and 1867, together with the equally popular six works in the later "Palliser" group that appeared between 1864 and 1880, are at the core of Trollope's fame. He is preeminent for his portrayal of the professional and landed classes in mid–Victorian England through his finely tuned sensitivity to the nuances of the complex class structure.

This aspect is prominent in *Dr. Thorne* where class tensions are an important factor in the plot as well as in the transactions between the doctor and his patients. Although Dr. Thorne is described in the opening sentence of this long novel as its "chief personage" (5) and later as "our hero" (20), the plot centers on the love between his niece, Mary, and Frank Gresham, the heir to the Greshambury estate. As the Greshams have fallen into debt, Frank is expected to marry a wealthy young woman so as to redeem the family's fortunes. Mary has no money, at least not until a sudden inheritance late in the novel that leads to its happy resolution. A further objection to Mary on the Greshams' part is her lack of an adequately lofty social status. The illegitimate daughter of Dr. Thorne's profligate brother, who was killed in a duel, she has been brought up by her uncle. She is gentle, kind, well educated, and good-looking, but her social level and her impecuniousness make her an unsuitable match for Frank in his parents' eyes.

The dubiousness of Mary's social status reflects also Dr. Thorne's own equivocal position in the class hierarchy. He is "a graduated physician"; this means that he had been educated at Oxford or Cambridge, and belongs to the uppermost tier of the mid–nineteenth-century British medical system. But even at that level his social standing is not high. He has the advantage of being related to a venerable old family in the area: "He was a second cousin to Mr. Thorne of Ullathorne, a Barsetshire squire living in the neighbourhood of Barchester, and who boasted that his estate had remained in his family, descending from Thorne to Thorne, longer than had been the case with any other estate or any other family in the county" (20–21). "But," Trollope immediately points out, "Dr. Thorne was only a second cousin; and, therefore, though he was entitled to talk of the blood as belonging to some extent to himself, he had no right to lay claim to any position in the county other than such as he might win for himself." In other words, he derives some social prestige from being distantly connected to the oldest family, but so distantly as not to enable him to command respect automatically by virtue of his "station" in the class hierarchy. For a doctor, family "connections," as they were called, were considered extremely important at a time when medical men were assessed by their manners, bearing, and appearance rather than by their actual professional expertise, which could be very hard for patients to judge, especially before the legal regulation of medicine and the institution of proper training. So Dr. Thorne is in the awkward position of being regarded by his landed patients as their social inferior. Yet they need his advice, they have on the whole a favorable opinion of his judgment and a certain grudging respect, even affection for him.

In the first selection, Dr. Thorne has aggravated the difficulties of his situation through his behavior and beliefs. After an early engagement in which he was jilted because of his brother's disreputable actions, he has remained a bachelor. This is seen as "a misfortune" (36) because a married man was thought to be more responsible. His appearance, too, is not as polished as was desirable ("rough though never dirty in his personal belongings"). But although he may be abrupt with "trifling ailments," he has an empathy amounting to tenderness for those genuinely in pain: apparently demanding, he is kindly when the occasion warrants. Dr. Thorne is perhaps too individualistic to be taken as the typical physician of the period. However, this figure does fulfill the traditional function of being a "confidential friend" to the families under his care; that phrase was coined by Worthington Hooker in his treatise, *Physician and Patient* (1849), to define the doctor's ideal relationship to his patients. Nineteenth-century literature abounds in doctors who, like Thorne, are wise family friends as well as medical attendants: Dr. Benassis in Honoré de Balzac's *Médecin de campagne* (1833; Country Doctor), Mr. Pratt in George's Eliot's story "Janet's Repentance" in *Scenes from Clerical Life* (1858), Dr. Kittredge in Oliver Wendell Holmes's *Elsie Venner* (1861), Mr. Gibson in Elizabeth Gaskell's *Wives and Daughters* (1866), and Dr. Ruhmschüttel in *Effi Briest* (1895) by the German novelist Theodor Fontane.

Yet *Dr. Thorne* also reveals many of the difficulties faced by doctors in the social reality of that time, notably as a result of the predominance of the class system within the profession too. For medical men were subject to a hierarchical order that had its own conventions at every level. By disregarding them Dr. Thorne reaps his fellow physicians' disapproval when he transgresses one of the unwritten rules of medical practice in mid-nineteenth-century Britain. Out of consideration for his patients' convenience Dr. Thorne himself dispenses medications ("common powders" and "vulgar ointments"), a task that was considered beneath the "dignity of a learned profession." While physicians prescribed medications, it was left to the much lower order of apothecaries (pharmacists) to do the actual "compounding," i.e., mixing, at a time when there were, of course, no prepackaged drugs. A physician, it was held, should use his head, not his hands; he should be "making experiments philosophically," that is, in a theoretical, speculative manner. Medical practice in *Dr. Thorne* clings to the old traditions. It is clear that the inhabitants of Barsetshire have by mid-century not heard of any of the advances in scientific medicine by then well underway, even though they are not far from London. For instance, Dr. Thorne is never shown using a stethoscope or any other instrument, or indeed doing anything beyond offering advice and dispensing medications. His method is to observe his patients closely, perhaps taking their pulse, but mainly he draws on his intimate familiarity with their family and medical history, their constitution and lifestyle as the basis for his treatment. He exemplifies a mode of practice that rested on the belief that the doctor's lengthy and extensive knowledge of the patient was the only reliable basis for good care.

The prime importance of social considerations in *Dr. Thorne* affords excellent insight into the intricacies of the doctor-patient relationship. On the one hand, patients are dependent on the doctor who knows them thoroughly. On the other hand, the doctor, is considered a social inferior, merely a paid employee; if his advice is uncongenial, he can readily be dismissed in favor of a more tractable successor, although the grave disadvantage to patients is then precisely the new doctor's scant acquaintance with their previous history. This problem is illustrated in two patients' interactions with Dr. Thorne: Lady Arabella and Sir Roger Scatcherd. While they differ in temperament and social position, the pattern of their association with Dr. Thorne is very similar.

In the second selection, Lady Arabella is an aristocrat who expects greater deference from Dr. Thorne than he is willing to grant her partly out of his independence of spirit, and partly because his Ullathorne connections raise his sense of his own worth. When Lady Arabella does not like his recommendations about the care of her series of sickly babies, she promptly switches to Dr. Thorne's rival, Dr. Fillgrave, who is more obsequious, but whose indulgence of Lady Arabella's wishes and whims proves disastrous. So she humbly returns to Dr. Thorne, recognizing the value of the cautious course of action he had advocated. He in turn is most generous in forgiving her temporary defection. Later on, when she is worried about having cancer, she again consults Dr. Thorne despite her reservations about his manner toward her. She faces a special quandary in wanting to keep Mary away from her son, Frank; she has to speak to Dr. Thorne about this tricky issue without so alienating him that he will withdraw from her his services that have become so necessary to her. This intertwining of medical and social matters leads to difficult challenges to the tact of both doctor and patient.

Even more than Lady Arabella, Sir Roger Scatcherd, in the third selection, sees Dr. Thorne as both his friend and his physician, although he is very torn in his feelings toward him. Dr. Thorne is a very special kind of friend on whom Sir Roger depends in various ways despite a lack of shared interests and occasional clashes. Sir Roger takes offense at the doctor's "severity" when Dr. Thorne tries to educate him about the dangers of drinking, an addiction that will soon kill him, the doctor warns. Dr. Thorne, who proves right in his admonitions and predictions, unquestionably has his patient's best interests at heart. Nevertheless, Sir

Roger is resentful of the unwelcome advice, and things come to a head in a crucial exchange that reveals the power conflicts between doctor and patient. For when Dr. Thorne staunchly asserts: "Scatcherd, I must do my duty to you, whether you like it or not," Sir Roger's immediate, scornful reply is: "That is to say, I am to pay you for trying to frighten me." The disagreement escalates into an open quarrel in which Sir Roger threatens to leave Dr. Thorne, a move that the doctor perspicaciously recognizes as "malicious vengeance." So Sir Roger resorts to the same tactic as Lady Arabella, doctor switching, when faced with disagreeable instructions, however sound they may be medically. Both envisage Dr. Thorne as their paid attendant, who is expected to give them not only respect and courtesy but also to endorse the conduct that pleases them. For the doctor to oppose their misguided wishes is taken as a personal affront to be remedied by changing to a more compliant physician.

Sir Roger's attitude toward Dr. Thorne is riddled with contradictions, summarized in the fact that the doctor is his only friend, yet one whom he dislikes. Their respective social levels are implicated in the tensions between them; for while Dr. Thorne is not rich, he is connected to the Thornes of Ullathorne, whereas Sir Roger is an upstart who has made a great deal of money and acquired his title only recently. This disparity does not prevent Sir Roger from demanding the same kind of deference as Lady Arabella, a hereditary aristocrat. Sir Roger's outbursts of temper, which may partly be attributable to his alcoholism, are in striking contrast to his wife's geniality to Dr. Thorne. "Lady Scatcherd and the doctor," we are told, "were on very familiar terms." To this troubled family Dr. Thorne is as much a friend as a physician.

Dr. Thorne's function as "confidential friend" to Sir Roger their previous discord notwithstanding, is confirmed in the scene when Sir Roger begs the doctor to be the sole executor of his estate and to assume charge of his only son (already an alcoholic in his twenties) after his own imminent death. These requests show the extent of Sir Roger's intimacy with Dr. Thorne as well as the wide range of demands that might be made on the family physician. Although Sir Roger's manner continues to be rather ungracious, there can be no doubt of his deep trust in his doctor.

Dr. Thorne's at times blunt directness is set in relief by the devious hypocrisy of his competitor, Dr. Fillgrave (the fourth selection). The name is patently satirical as is also the physical description of this short, plump man who aspires by every means at his disposal to acquire an air likely to impress his patients. Dr. Fillgrave is vain, pompous, and jubilant at the prospect of displacing Dr. Thorne as physician to Sir Roger, the richest man in the area. His greed and his self-importance become apparent when Sir Roger calls him in after one of his periodic altercations with Dr. Thorne. On his arrival, however, Dr. Fillgrave is annoyed at being kept waiting for he considers this a sign of disrespect for him. And when he hears that Sir Roger, having recovered from his hangover, no longer wants medical attention at all, he is as much offended at the loss of prestige as disappointed at the loss of the fee he had eagerly expected. Since he has not rendered any medical services, should Dr. Fillgrave accept the generous honorarium Lady Scatcherd offers to appease him and get rid of him, or is he morally obliged to refuse it? Fillgrave's urge to gratify his greed here comes into conflict with the sententious pronouncements he had made earlier in the novel about the duty of doctors to stand above financial rewards. The comedy of the negotiations between him and Lady Scatcherd is intensified when Dr. Thorne unsuspectingly arrives to visit his patient, who had failed to inform him that he was carrying out his threat to switch doctors. Fillgrave grows increasingly furious as he tries, unsuccessfully, to maintain a dignified front even as he pours scorn on his rival. This ludicrous scene closes, fittingly, with Lady Scatcherd's revelation that she had slipped Fillgrave's payment into his hat during his "tantrum." The very word "tantrum," by suggesting childish behavior, carries an oblique condemnation of Fillgrave's conduct.

This grotesque episode has a number of implications. First of all, it underscores Dr. Thorne's consistent honesty in contrast to Fillgrave's self-seeking hypocrisy. Thorne's nobility and devotion to his patients, however cantakerous they may be, is brought out by Fillgrave's pretentiousness and concern with his own image and well-being. Secondly, the importance of money in the transactions between doctors and patients is made very clear. The idealistic Thorne charges modest fees and leads a simple, almost spartan life, whereas the materialistic Fillgrave is more interested in rich pickings such as the kind of carriage he rides in than in the patient's health. The contrast between the two may be rather extreme, but it serves to show the great spectrum of attitudes motivating practitioners. To Fillgrave money is a question of status, a symbol of the esteem in which he wants to be held. Although an unavoidable element in the interface between doctors and patients, money is here depicted as a disturbing factor that may impinge negatively on the therapeutic alliance.

The combination of social class and financial considerations made the practice of medicine in the mid-nineteenth century a tricky enterprise that required incessant tact on the doctor's part if he was to succeed in steering patients toward the course best for their health without alienating them. The primitiveness of the interventions available before scientific advances became widely diffused made the physician's task much harder. As a "confidential friend" he had to rely on the persuasive force of his personality and on the trust he could inspire. Dr. Thorne is largely able to fulfill that role, but not without setbacks and the input of enormous efforts of benevolence and wisdom that are sometimes spurned.

Dr. Thorne offers a valuable baseline image of medical practice before it became a science; it reveals the precariousness of the physician's position from both the medical and social perspectives. The type of action that Dr. Thorne recommends to his patients is decided by his subjective impressions of their condition, by his experience of their personal and family history, and by sheer common sense (e.g., not to abuse alcohol). Trollope's novel provides today's readers with a surprising picture of the complexities involved in medicine as an intuitive art rather than a scientific endeavor, and it also shows vividly the constraints imposed on the doctor by the social realities in which he was embedded. Dr. Thorne is criticized on the one hand for being too "democratic" and for charging low fees and on the other hand for asserting his opinions instead of pandering to his patients. Compared to our own time, the differences are striking. Patients, by holding the purse-strings, exercised decisive power; were they able to do so wisely? Was the mingling of the personal and the social with the medical relationship beneficial to either patients or doctors? How should tricky decisions about the best course of treatment be made? Does the social reality of today's managed care create predicaments as pressing as those faced by Dr. Thorne? Is money, i.e., affordability, still as crucial as in Trollope's day?

Dr. Thorne

Anthony Trollope

And thus Dr Thorne became settled for life in the little village of Greshamsbury. As was then the wont with many country practitioners, and as should be the wont with them all if they consulted their own dignity a little less and the comforts of their customers somewhat more, he added the business of a dispensing apothecary to that of physician. In doing so, he was of course much reviled. Many people around him declared that he could not truly be a doctor, or, at any rate, a doctor to be so called; and his brethren in the art living around him, though they knew that his diplomas, degrees, and certificates were all *en règle* (in good order) rather countenanced the report. There was much about this newcomer which did not endear him to his own profession. In the first place he was a new-comer, and, as such, was of course to be regarded by other doctors as being *de trop* (superfluous). Greshamsbury was only fifteen miles from Barchester, where there was a regular depot of medical skill, and but eight from Silverbridge, where a properly established physician had been in residence for the last forty years. Dr Thorne's predecessor at Greshamsbury had been a humble-minded general practitioner, gifted with a due respect for the physicians of the county; and he, though he had been allowed to physic the servants, and sometimes the children

From Anthony Trollope, *Dr. Thorne* (New York: Penguin, 1991), pp. 31–32, 34–35, 35–36.

at Greshamsbury, had never had the presumption to put himself on a par with his betters.

Then, also, Dr Thorne, though a graduated physician, though entitled beyond all dispute to call himself a doctor, according to all the laws of the colleges, made it known to the East Barsetshire world, very soon after he had seated himself at Greshamsbury, that his rate of pay was to be seven-and-sixpence a visit within a circuit of five miles, with a proportionately increased charge at proportionately increased distances. Now there was something low, mean, unprofessional, and democratic in this; so, at least, said the children of Esculapius [the Roman god of medicine] gathered together in conclave at Barchester. In the first place, it showed that this Thorne was always thinking of his money, like an apothecary, as he was; whereas, it would have behoved him, as a physician, had he had the feelings of a physician under his hat, to have regarded his own pursuits in a purely philosophical spirit, and to have taken any gain which might have accrued as an accidental adjunct to his station in life. A physician should take his fee without letting his left hand know what his right hand was doing; it should be taken without a thought, without a look, without a move of the facial muscles; the true physician should hardly be aware that the last friendly grasp of the hand had been made more precious by the touch of gold. Whereas, that fellow Thorne would lug out half a crown from his breeches pocket and give it in change for a ten-shilling piece. And then it was clear that this man had no appreciation of the dignity of a learned profession. He might constantly be seen compounding medicines in the shop, at the left hand of his front door; not making experiments philosophically in materia medica for the benefit of coming ages—which, if he did, he should have done in the seclusion of his study, far from profane eyes—but positively putting together common powders for rural bowels, or spreading vulgar ointments for agricultural ailments.

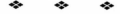

He had, moreover, other difficulties to encounter in his professional career. It was something in his favour that he understood his business; something that he was willing to labour at it with energy; and resolved to labour at it conscientiously. He had also other gifts, such as conversational brilliancy, an aptitude for true good fellowship, firmness in friendship, and general honesty of disposition, which stood him in stead as he advanced in life. But, at his first starting, much that belonged to himself personally was against him. Let him enter what house he would, he entered it with a conviction, often expressed to himself, that he was equal as a man to the proprietor, equal as a human being to the proprietress. To age he would allow deference, and to special recognised talent—at least, so he said; to rank, also, he would pay that respect which was its clear recognised prerogative; he would let a lord walk out of a room before him if he did not happen to forget it; in speaking to a duke he would address him as his Grace; and he would in no way assume a familiarity with bigger men than himself, allowing to the bigger man the privilege of making the first advances. But beyond this he would admit that no man should walk the earth with head higher than his own.

He did not talk of these things much; he offended no rank by boasts of his own equality; he did not absolutely tell the Earl de Courcy in words, that the privilege of dining at Courcy Castle was to him no greater than the privilege of dining at Courcy Parsonage; but there was that in his manner that told it. The feeling in itself was perhaps good, and was certainly much justified by the manner in which he bore himself to those below him in rank; but there was folly in the resolution to run counter to the world's recognised rules on such matters; and much absurdity in his mode of doing so, seeing that at heart he was a thorough Conservative. It is hardly too much to say that he naturally hated a lord at first sight; but, nevertheless, he would have expended his means, his blood, and spirit, in fighting for the upper house of Parliament.

Such a disposition, until it was thoroughly understood, did not tend to ingratiate him with the wives of the country gentlemen among whom he had to look for practice. And then, also, there was not much in his individual manner to recommend him to the favour of ladies. He was brusque, authoritative, given to contradiction, rough though never dirty in his personal belongings, and inclined to indulge in a sort of quiet raillery, which sometimes was not thoroughly understood. People did not always know whether he was laughing at them or with them; and some people were, perhaps, inclined to think that a doctor should not laugh at all when called in to act doctorially.

When he was known, indeed, when the core of the fruit had been reached, when the huge proportions of that loving, trusting heart had been learned, and understood, and appreciated, when that honesty had been recognised, that manly, and almost womanly tenderness had been felt, then, indeed, the doctor was acknowledged to be adequate to his profession. To trifling ailments he was too often brusque. Seeing that he accepted money for the cure of such, he should, we may say, have cured them without an offensive manner. So far he is without defence. But to real suffering no one found him brusque; no patient lying painfully on a bed of sickness ever thought him rough.

Lady Arabella, a Patient in Two Minds

Anthony Trollope

Dr Thorne's pretensions, mixed with his subversive professional democratic tendencies, his seven-and-sixpenny visits, added to his utter disregard of Lady Arabella's airs, were too much for her spirit. He brought Frank [her son] through his first troubles, and that at first ingratiated her; he was equally successful with the early dietary of Augusta and Beatrice [her daughters]; but, as his success obtained in direct opposition to the Courcy Castle nursery principles, this hardly did much in his favour. When the third daughter was born, he at once declared that she was a very weakly flower, and sternly forbade the mother to go to London. The mother, loving her babe, obeyed; but did not the less hate the doctor for the order, which she firmly believed was given at the instance and express dictation of Mr Gresham. Then another little girl came into the world, and the doctor was more imperative than ever as to the nursery rules and the excellence of country air. Quarrels were thus engendered, and Lady Arabella was taught to believe that this doctor of her husband's was after all no Solomon. In her husband's absence she sent for Dr Fillgrave, giving very express intimation that he would not have to wound either his eyes or dignity by encountering his enemy; and she found Dr Fillgrave a great comfort to her.

Then Dr Thorne gave Mr Gresham to understand that, under such circumstances, he could not visit professionally at Greshamsbury any longer.

From Anthony Trollope, *Dr. Thorne* (New York: Penguin, 1991), pp. 38–39, 162, 169.

The poor squire saw there was no help for it, and though he still maintained his friendly connexion with his neighbour, the seven-and-sixpenny visits were at an end. Dr Fillgrave from Barchester, and the gentleman at Silverbridge, divided the responsibility between them, and the nursery principles of Courcy Castle were again in vogue at Greshamsbury.

So things went on for years, and those years were years of sorrow. We must not ascribe to our doctor's enemies the sufferings, and sickness, and deaths that occurred. The four frail little ones that died would probably have been taken had Lady Arabella been more tolerant of Dr Thorne. But the fact was, that they did die; and that the mother's heart then got the better of the woman's pride, and Lady Arabella humbled herself before Dr Thorne. She humbled herself, or would have done so, had the doctor permitted her. But he, with his eyes full of tears, stopped the utterance of her apology, took her two hands in his, pressed them warmly, and assured her that his joy in returning would be great, for the love that he bore to all that belonged to Greshamsbury. And so the seven-and-sixpenny visits were recommenced; and the great triumph of Dr Fillgrave came to an end.

Great was the joy in the Greshamsbury nursery when the second change took place. Among the doctor's attributes, not hitherto mentioned, was an aptitude for the society of children. He delighted to talk to children, and to play with them. He would carry them on his back, three or four at a time, roll with them on the ground, race with them in the gardens, invent games for them, contrive amusements in circumstances which seemed quite adverse to all manner of delight; and, above all, his physic was not nearly so nasty as that which came from Silverbridge.

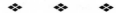

The Lady Arabella, though she was not personally attached to the doctor with quite so much warmth as some others of her family, still had reasons of her own for not dispensing with his visits to the house. She was one of his patients, and a patient fearful of the disease with which she was threatened. Though she thought the doctor to be arrogant, deficient as to properly submissive demeanour towards herself, an instigator to marital parsimony in her lord, one altogether opposed to herself and her interests in Greshamsbury politics, nevertheless, she did feel trust in him as a medical man. She had no wish to be rescued out of his hands by any Dr Fillgrave, as regarded that complaint of hers, much as she may have desired, and did desire, to sever him from all Greshamsbury councils in all matters not touching the healing art.

Now the complaint of which the Lady Arabelia was afraid, was cancer: and her only present confidant in this matter was Dr Thorne.

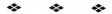

Lady Arabella resolved to open her mind to the doctor, and to make it
intelligible to him that, under present circumstances, Mary's visits at
Greshamsbury had better be discontinued. She would have given much,
however, to have escaped this business. She had in her time tried one or
two falls with the doctor, and she was conscious that she had never yet
got the better of him: and then she was in a slight degree afraid of Mary
herself. She had a presentiment that it would not be so easy to banish
Mary from Greshamsbury: she was not sure that that young lady would
not boldly assert her right to her place in the schoolroom; appeal loudly
to the squire, and, perhaps, declare her determination of marrying the
heir, out before them all. The squire would be sure to uphold her in
that, or in anything else.

And then, too, there would be the greatest difficulty in wording her
request to the doctor; and Lady Arabella was sufficiently conscious of her
own weakness to know that she was not always very good at words. But
the doctor, when hard pressed, was never at fault: he could say the
bitterest things in the quietest tone, and Lady Arabella had a great dread
of these bitter things. What, also, if he should desert her himself; withdraw from her his skill and knowledge of her bodily wants and ailments
now that he was so necessary to her?

Sir Roger, a Cantakerous Patient

Anthony Trollope

Scatcherd had but one friend in the world. And, indeed, this friend was no friend in the ordinary acceptance of the word. He neither ate with him nor drank with him, nor even frequently talked with him. Their pursuits in life were wide asunder. Their tastes were all different. The society in which each moved very seldom came together. Scatcherd had nothing in unison with this solitary friend; but he trusted him, and he trusted no other living creature on God's earth.

He trusted this man; but even him he did not trust thoroughly; not at least as one friend should trust another. He believed that this man would not rob him; would probably not lie to him; would not endeavour to make money of him; would not count him up or speculate on him, and make out a balance of profit and loss; and, therefore, he determined to use him. But he put no trust whatever in his friend's counsel, in his modes of thought; none in his theory, and none in his practice. He disliked his friend's counsel, and, in fact, disliked his society, for his friend was somewhat apt to speak to him in a manner approaching to severity. Now Roger Scatcherd had done many things in the world, and made much money; whereas his friend had done but few things, and made no money. It was not to be endured that the practical, efficient man should be taken to task by the man who proved himself to be

From Anthony Trollope, *Dr. Thorne* (New York: Penguin, 1991), pp. 113–114, 116–120.

neither practical nor efficient; not to be endured, certainly, by Roger Scatcherd, who looked on men of his own class as the men of the day, and on himself as by no means the least among them.

The friend was our friend Dr Thorne.

The doctor's first acquaintance with Scatcherd has been already explained. He was necessarily thrown into communication with the man at the time of the trial [of his brother], and Scatcherd then had not only sufficient sense, but sufficient feeling also to know that the doctor behaved very well. This communication had in different ways been kept up between them. Soon after the trial Scatcherd had begun to rise, and his first savings had been intrusted to the doctor's care. This had been the beginning of a pecuniary connexion which had never wholly ceased, and which had led to the purchase of Boxall Hill, and to the loan of large sums of money to the squire.

In another way also there had been a close alliance between them, and one not always of a very pleasant description. The doctor was, and long had been, Sir Roger's medical attendant, and, in his unceasing attempts to rescue the drunkard from the fate which was so much to be dreaded, he not unfrequently was driven into a quarrel with his patient.

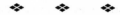

Lady Scatcherd and the doctor were on very familiar terms as regarded her little domestic inconveniences.

'Tell Sir Roger I am here, will you?' said the doctor.

'You'll take a drop of sherry before you go up?' said the lady.

'Not a drop, thank you,' said the doctor.

'Or, perhaps, a little cordial?'

'Not a drop of anything, thank you; I never do, you know.'

'Just a thimbleful of this?' said the lady, producing from some recess under the sideboard a bottle of brandy; 'just a thimbleful? It's what he takes himself.'

When Lady Scatcherd found that even this argument failed, she led the way to the great man's bedroom.

'Well, doctor! well, doctor! well, doctor!' was the greeting with which our son of Galen [famous doctor of antiquity] was saluted some time before he entered the sick-room. His approaching step was heard, and thus the *ci-devant* (former) Barchester stonemason saluted his coming friend. The voice was loud and powerful, but not clear and sonorous. What voice that is nurtured on brandy can ever be clear? It had about it a peculiar huskiness, a dissipated guttural tone, which Thorne immediately recognised, and recognised as being more marked, more guttural, and more husky than heretofore.

'So you've smelt me out, have you, and come for your fee? Ha! ha! ha! Well, I have had a sharpish bout of it, as her ladyship there no doubt has told you. Let her alone to make the worst of it. But, you see, you're too late, man. I've bilked the old gentleman again, without troubling you.'

'Any way, I'm glad you're something better, Scatcherd.'

'Something! I don't know what you call something. I never was better in my life. Ask Winterbones [the clerk] there.'

'Indeed, now, Scatcherd, you ain't; you're bad enough if you only knew it. And as for Winterbones, he has no business here up in your bedroom, which stinks of gin so, it does. Don't you believe him, doctor; he ain't well, nor yet nigh well.'

Winterbones, when the above ill-natured allusion was made to the aroma coming from his libations, might be seen to deposit surreptitiously beneath the little table at which he sat, the cup with which he had performed them.

The doctor, in the meantime, had taken Sir Roger's hand on the pretext of feeling his pulse, but was drawing quite as much information from the touch of the sick man's skin, and the look of the sick man's eye.

'I think Mr Winterbones had better go back to the London office,' said he. 'Lady Scatcherd will be your best clerk for some little time, Sir Roger.'

'Then I'll be d—if Mr Winterbones does anything of the kind,' said he; 'so there's an end of that.'

'Very well,' said the doctor. 'A man can die but once. It is my duty to suggest measures for putting off the ceremony as long as possible. Perhaps, however, you may wish to hasten it.'

'Well, I am not very anxious about it, one way or the other,' said Scatcherd. And as he spoke there came a fierce gleam from his eye, which seemed to say—'If that's the bugbear with which you wish to frighten me, you will find that you are mistaken.'

'Now, doctor, don't let him talk that way, don't,' said Lady Scatcherd, with her handkerchief to her eyes.

'Now, my lady, do you cut it; cut at once,' said Sir Roger, turning hastily round to his better-half; and his better-half, knowing that the province of a woman is to obey, did cut it. But as she went she gave the doctor a pull by the coat sleeve, so that thereby his healing faculties might be sharpened to the very utmost.

'The best woman in the world, doctor; the very best,' said he, as the door closed behind the wife of his bosom.

'I'm sure of it,' said the doctor.

'Yes, till you find a better one,' said Scatcherd. 'Ha! ha! ha! but good or bad, there are some things which a woman can't understand, and some things which she ought not to be let to understand.'

'It's natural she should be anxious about your health, you know.'

'I don't know that,' said the contractor. 'She'll be very well off. All that whining won't keep a man alive, at any rate.'

There then was a pause, during which the doctor continued his medical examination. To this the patient submitted with a bad grace, but still he did submit.

'We must turn over a new leaf Sir Roger; indeed we must.'

'Bother,' said Sir Roger.

'Well, Scatcherd; I must do my duty to you, whether you like it or not.'

'That is to say, I am to pay you for trying to frighten me.'

'No human nature can stand such shocks as these much longer.'

'Winterbones,' said the contractor, turning to his clerk, 'go down, go down, I say; but don't be out of the way. If you go to the public-house, by G—, you may stay there for me. When I take a drop,—that is if I ever do, it does not stand in the way of work.' So Mr Winterbones, picking up his cup again, and concealing it in some way beneath his coat flap, retreated out of the room, and the two friends were alone.

'Scatcherd,' said the doctor, 'you have been as near your God, as any man ever was who afterwards ate and drank in this world.'

'Have I, now?' said the railway hero, apparently somewhat startled.

'Indeed you have; indeed you have.'

'And now I'm all right again?'

'All right! How can you be all right, when you know that your limbs refuse to carry you? All right! why the blood is still beating round your brain with a violence that would destroy any other brain but yours.'

'Ha! ha! ha!' laughed Scatcherd. He was very proud of thinking himself to be differently organised from other men. 'Ha! ha! ha! Well, and what am I to do now?'

The whole of the doctor's prescription we will not give at length. To some of his ordinances Sir Roger promised obedience; to others he objected violently, and to one or two he flatly refused to listen. The great stumbling-block was this, that total abstinence from business for two weeks was enjoined; and that it was impossible, so Sir Roger said, that he should abstain for two days.

'If you work,' said the doctor, 'in your present state, you will certainly have recourse to the stimulus of drink; and if you drink, most assuredly you will die.'

'Stimulus! Why, do you think I can't work without Dutch courage?'

'Scatcherd, I know that there is brandy in the room at this moment, and that you have been taking it within these two hours.'

'You smell that fellow's gin,' said Scatcherd.

'I feel the alcohol working within your veins,' said the doctor, who still had his hand on his patient's arm.

Sir Roger turned himself roughly in the bed so as to get away from his Mentor, and then he began to threaten in his turn.

'I'll tell you what it is, doctor; I've made up my mind, and I'll do it. I'll send for Fillgrave.'

'Very well,' said he of Greshamsbury, 'send for Filigrave. Your case is one in which even he can hardly go wrong.'

'You think you can hector me, and do as you like because you had me under your thumb in other days. You're a very good fellow, Thorne, but I ain't sure that you are the best doctor in all England.'

'You may be sure I am not; you may take me for the worst if you will. But while I am here as your medical adviser, I can only tell you the truth to the best of my thinking. Now the truth is this, that another bout of drinking will in all probability kill you; and any recourse to stimulus in your present condition may do so.'

'I'll send for Fillgrave—'

'Well, send for Fillgrave, only do it at once. Believe me at any rate in this, that whatever you do, you should do at once. Oblige me in this; let Lady Scatcherd take away that brandy bottle till Dr Fillgrave comes.'

'I'm d—if I do. Do you think I can't have a bottle of brandy in my room without swigging?'

'I think you'll be less likely to swig it if you can't get at it.'

Sir Roger made another angry turn in his bed as well as his half-paralysed limbs would let him; and then, after a few moments' peace, renewed his threats with increased violence.

'Yes; I'll have Fillgrave over here. If a man be ill, really ill, he should have the best advice he can get. I'll have Fillgrave, and I'll have that other fellow from Silverbridge to meet him. What's his name?—Century.'

The doctor turned his head away; for though the occasion was serious, he could not help smiling at the malicious vengeance with which his friend proposed to gratify himself.

'I will; and Rerechild too. What's the expense? I suppose five or six pound apiece will do it; eh, Thorne?'

'Oh, yes; that will be liberal I should say. But, Sir Roger, will you allow me to suggest what you ought to do? I don't know how far you may be joking—'

'Joking!' shouted the baronet; 'you tell a man he's dying and joking in the same breath. You'll find I'm not joking.'

'Well, I dare say not. But if you have not full confidence in me—'

'I have no confidence in you at all.'

'Then why not send to London? Expense is no object to you.'

'It is an object; a great object.'

'Nonsense! Send to London for Sir Omicron Pie: send for some man whom you will really trust when you see him.'

'There's not one of the lot I'd trust as soon as Fillgrave. I've known Fillgrave all my life, and I trust him. I'll send for Fillgrave and put my case in his hands. If any one can do anything for me, Fillgrave is the man.

'Then in God's name send for Fillgrave,' said the doctor. 'And now goodbye, Scatcherd; and as you do send for him, give him a fair chance. Do not destroy yourself by more brandy before he comes.'

'That's my affair, and his; not yours,' said the patient.

'So be it: give me your hand, at any rate, before I go. I wish you well through it, and when you are well, I'll come and see you.'

'Good-bye—good-bye; and look here, Thorne, you'll be talking to Lady Scatcherd downstairs, I know; now, no nonsense. You understand me, eh? no nonsense, you know.'

Dr. Fillgrave, a Rival

Anthony Trollope

The doctor, that is our doctor, had thought nothing more of the message which had been sent to that other doctor, Dr Fillgrave; nor in truth did the baronet. Lady Scatcherd had thought of it, but her husband during the rest of the day was not in a humour which allowed her to remind him that he would soon have a new physician on his hands; so she left the difficulty to arrange itself, waiting in some little trepidation till Dr Fillgrave should show himself.

It was well that Sir Roger was not dying for want of his assistance, for when the message reached Barchester, Dr Fillgrave was some five or six miles out of town, at Plumptead; and as he did not get back till late in the evening, he felt himself necessitated to put off his visit to Boxall Hill till the next morning. Had he chanced to have been made acquainted with that little conversation about the pump, he would probably have postponed it even yet a while longer.

He was, however, by no means sorry to be summoned to the bedside of Sir Roger Scatcherd. It was well known at Barchester, and very well known to Dr Fillgrave, that Sir Roger and Dr Thorne were old friends. It was very well known to him also, that Sir Roger, in all his bodily ailments, had hitherto been contented to entrust his safety to the skill of his old friend. Sir Roger was in his way a great man, and much

From Anthony Trollope, *Dr. Thorne* (New York: Penguin, 1991), pp. 140–147, 148–151.

58

talked of in Barchester, and rumour had already reached the ears of the Barchester Galen, that the great railway contractor was ill. When, therefore, he received a peremptory summons to go over to Boxall Hill, he could not but think that some pure light had broken in upon Sir Roger's darkness, and taught him at last where to look for true medical accomplishment.

And then, also, Sir Roger was the richest man in the county, and to county practitioners a new patient with large means is a godsend; how much greater a godsend when he be not only acquired, but taken also from some rival practitioner, need hardly be explained.

Dr Fillgrave, therefore, was somewhat elated when, after a very early breakfast, he stepped into the post-chaise which was to carry him to Boxall Hill. Dr Fillgrave's professional advancement had been sufficient to justify the establishment of a brougham, in which he paid his ordinary visits round Barchester; but this was a special occasion, requiring special speed, and about to produce no doubt a special guerdon, and therefore a pair of post-horses were put in to request.

It was hardly yet nine when the post-boy somewhat loudly rang the bell at Sir Roger's door; and then Dr Fillgrave, for the first time, found himself in the new grand hall of Boxall Hill House.

'I'll tell my lady,' said the servant, showing him into the grand dining-room; and there for some fifteen or twenty minutes Dr Fillgrave walked up and down the length of the Turkey carpet all alone.

Dr Fillgrave was not a tall man, and was perhaps rather more inclined to corpulence than became his height. In his stockingfeet, according to the usually received style of measurement, he was five feet five; and he had a little round abdominal protuberance, which an inch and a half added to the heels of his boots hardly enabled him to carry off as well as he himself would have wished. Of this he was apparently conscious, and it gave to him an air of not being entirely at his ease. There was, however, a personal dignity in his demeanour, a propriety in his gait, and an air of authority in his gestures which should prohibit one from stigmatizing those efforts at altitude as a failure. No doubt he did achieve much; but, nevertheless, the effort would occasionally betray itself, and the story of the frog and the ox would irresistibly force itself into one's mind at those moments when it most behoved Dr Fillgrave to be magnificent.

But if the bulgy roundness of his person and the shortness of his legs in any way detracted from his personal importance these trifling defects were, he was well aware, more than atoned for by the peculiar dignity of his countenance. If his legs were short, his face was not; if there was any undue preponderance below the waistcoat, all was in due symmetry above the necktie. His hair was grey, not grizzled nor white, but properly grey; and stood up straight from off his temples on each side with an unbending determination of purpose. His whiskers, which were of an admirable shape, coming down and turning gracefully at the angle of his jaw, were grey also, but somewhat darker than his hair. His enemies in Barchester declared that their perfect shade was produced by a leaden comb. His eyes were not brilliant, but were very effective, and well under command. He was rather short-sighted, and a pair of eye-glasses was always on his nose, or in his hand. His nose was long, and well pronounced, and his chin, also, was sufficiently prominent; but the great feature of his face was his mouth. The amount of secret medical knowledge of which he could give assurance by the pressure of those lips was truly wonderful. By his lips, also, he could be most exquisitely courteous, or most sternly forbidding. And not only could he be either the one or the other; but he could at his will assume any shade of difference between the two, and produce any mixture of sentiment.

When Dr Fillgrave was first shown into Sir Roger's diningroom, he walked up and down the room for a while with easy, jaunty step, with his hands joined together behind his back, calculating the price of the furniture, and counting the heads which might be adequately entertained in a room of such noble proportions; but in seven or eight minutes an air of impatience might have been seen to suffuse his face. Why could he not be shown up into the sick man's room? What necessity could there be for keeping him there, as though he were some apothecary with a box of leeches in his pocket? He then rang the bell, perhaps a little violently. 'Does Sir Roger know that I am here?' he said to the servant. 'I'll tell my lady,' said the man, again vanishing.

For five minutes more he walked up and down, calculating no longer the value of the furniture, but rather that of his own importance. He was not wont to be kept waiting in this way; and though Sir Roger Scatcherd was at present a great and a rich man, Dr Fillgrave had remembered him a very small and a very poor man. He now began to think of Sir Roger as the stone-mason, and to chafe somewhat more violently at being so kept by such a man.

When one is impatient, five minutes is as the duration of all time, and a quarter of an hour is eternity. At the end of twenty minutes the step of Dr Fillgrave up and down the room had become very quick, and he had just made up his mind that he would not stay there all day to the serious detriment, perhaps fatal injury, of his other expectant patients. His hand was again on the bell, and was about to be used with vigour, when the door opened and Lady Scatcherd entered.

The door opened and Lady Scatcherd entered; but she did so very slowly, as though she were afraid to come into her own dining-room. We must go back a little and see how she had been employed during those twenty minutes.

'Oh laws!' Such had been her first exclamation on hearing that the doctor was in the diningroom. She was standing at the time with her housekeeper in a small room in which she kept her linen and jam, and in which, in company with the same housekeeper, she spent the happiest moments of her life.

'Oh laws! now, Hannah, what shall we do?'

'Send 'un up at once to the master, my lady! let John take 'un up.

'There'll be such a row in the house,—Hannah; I know there will.'

'But surely didn't he send for 'un? Let the master have the row himself, then; that's what I'd do, my lady,' added Hannah, seeing that her ladyship still stood trembling in doubt, biting her thumb-nail.

'You couldn't go up to the master yourself, could you now, Hannah?' said Lady Scatcherd in her most persuasive tone.

'Why no,' said Hannah, after a little deliberation; 'no, I'm afeard I couldn't.'

'Then I must just face it myself.' And up went the wife to tell her lord that the physician for whom he had sent had come to—attend his bidding.

In the interview which then took place the baronet had not indeed been violent, but he had been very determined. Nothing on earth, he said, should induce him to see Dr Fillgrave and offend his dear old friend Thorne.

'But, Roger,' said her ladyship, half crying, or rather pretending to cry in her vexation, 'what shall I do with the man? How shall I get him out of the house?'

'Put him under the pump,' said the baronet; and he laughed his peculiar low guttural laugh, which told so plainly of the havoc which brandy had made in his throat.

'That's nonsense, Roger; you know I can't put him under the pump. Now you are ill, and you'd better see him just for five minutes. I'll make it all right with Dr Thorne.'

'I'll be d—if I do, my lady.' All the people about Boxall Hill called poor Lady Scatcherd 'my lady,' as if there was some excellent joke in it; and so, indeed, there was.

'You know you needn't mind nothing he says, nor yet take nothing he sends: and I'll tell him not to come no more. Now do'ee see him, Roger.'

But there was no coaxing Roger over now, or indeed ever: he was a wilful, headstrong, masterful man; a tyrant always, though never a cruel one; and accustomed to rule his wife and household as despotically as he did his gangs of workmen. Such men it is not easy to coax over.

'You go down and tell him I don't want him, and won't see him, and that's an end of it. If he chose to earn his money, why didn't he come yesterday when he was sent for? I'm well now, and don't want him; and what's more, I won't have him. Winterbones, lock the door.'

So Winterbones, who during this interview had been at work at his little table, got up to lock the door, and Lady Scatcherd had no alternative but to pass through it before the last edict was obeyed.

Lady Scatcherd, with slow step, went downstairs and again sought counsel with Hannah, and the two, putting their heads together, agreed that the only cure for the present evil was to be found in a good fee. So Lady Scatcherd, with a five-pound note in her hand, and trembling in every limb, went forth to encounter the august presence of Dr Fillgrave.

As the door opened, Dr Fillgrave dropped the bell-rope which was in his hand, and bowed low to the lady. Those who knew the doctor well, would have known from his bow that he was not well pleased; it was as much as though he said, 'Lady Scatcherd, I am your most obedient humble servant; at any rate it appears that it is your pleasure to treat me as such.'

Lady Scatcherd did not understand all this; but she perceived at once that the man was angry.

'I hope Sir Roger does not find himself worse,' said the doctor. 'The morning is getting on; shall I step up and see him?'

'Hem! ha! oh! Why, you see, Dr Fillgrave, Sir Roger finds hisself vastly better this morning, vastly so.'

'I'm very glad to hear it, very; but as the morning is getting on, shall I step up to see Sir Roger?'

'Why, Dr Fillgrave, sir, you see he finds hisself so much hisself this morning, that he a'most thinks it would be a shame to trouble you.'

'A shame to trouble me!' This was a sort of shame which Dr. Fillgrave did not at all comprehend. 'A shame to trouble me! Why, Lady Scatcherd—'

Lady Scatcherd saw that she had nothing for it but to make the whole matter intelligible. Moreover, seeing that she appreciated more thoroughly the smallness of Dr Fillgrave's person than she did the peculiar greatness of his demeanour, she began to be a shade less afraid of him than she had thought she should have been.

'Yes, Dr Fillgrave; you see, when a man like he gets well, he can't abide the idea of doctors: now yesterday, he was all for sending for you; but today he comes to hisself, and don't seem to want no doctor at all.'

Then did Dr Fillgrave seem to grow out of his boots, so suddenly did he take upon himself sundry modes of expansive attitude;—to grow out of his boots and to swell upwards, till his angry eyes almost looked down on Lady Scatcherd, and each erect hair bristled up towards the heavens.

'This is very singular, very singular, Lady Scatcherd; very singular, indeed; very singular; quite unusual. I have come here from Barchester, at some considerable inconvenience, at some very considerable inconvenience, I may say, to my regular patients; and—and—and—I don't know that anything so very singular ever occurred to me before.' And then Dr Fillgrave, with a compression of his lips which almost made the poor woman sink into the ground, moved towards the door.

Then Lady Scatcherd bethought her of her great panacea. 'It isn't about the money, you know, doctor,' said she; 'of course Sir Roger don't expect you to come here with posthorses for nothing.' In this, by the by, Lady Scatcherd did not stick quite close to veracity, for Sir Roger, had he known it, would by no means have assented to any payment; and the note which her ladyship held in her hand was taken from her own private purse. 'It ain't at all about the money, doctor;' and then she tendered the bank-note, which she thought would immediately make all things smooth.

Now Dr Fillgrave dearly loved a five-pound fee. What physician is so unnatural as not to love it? He dearly loved a five-pound fee; but he loved his dignity better. He was angry also; and like all angry men, he loved his grievance. He felt that he had been badly treated; but if he took the money he would throw away his right to indulge any such feeling. At that moment his outraged dignity and his cherished anger were worth more to him than a five-pound note. He looked at it with wishful but still averted eyes, and then sternly refused the tender.

'No, madam,' said he; 'no, no;' and with his right hand raised with his eye-glasses in it, he motioned away the tempting paper. 'No; I should have been happy to have given Sir Roger the benefit of any medical skill I may have, seeing that I was specially called in—'

'But, doctor; if the man's well, you know—'

'Oh, of course; if he's well, and does not choose to see me, there's an end of it. Should he have any relapse, as my time is valuable, he will perhaps oblige me by sending elsewhere. Madam, good morning. I will, if you will allow me, ring for my carriage—that is, post-chaise.'

'But, doctor, you'll take the money; you must take the money; indeed you'll take the money,' said Lady Scatcherd, who had now become really unhappy at the idea that her husband's unpardonable whim had brought this man with post-horses all the way from Barchester, and that he was to be paid nothing for his time nor costs.

'No, madam, no. I could not think of it. Sir Roger, I have no doubt, will know better another time. It is not a question of money; not at all.'

'But it is a question of money, doctor; and you really shall, you must.' And poor Lady Scatcherd, in her anxiety to acquit herself at any rate of any pecuniary debt to the doctor, came to personal close quarters with him, with the view of forcing the note into his hands.

'Quite impossible, quite impossible,' said the doctor, still cherishing his grievance, and valiantly rejecting the root of all evil. 'I shall not do anything of the kind, Lady Scatcherd.'

'Now doctor, do'ee; to oblige me.'

'Quite out of the question.' And so, with his hands and hat behind his back, in token of his utter refusal to accept any pecuniary accommodation of his injury, he made his way backwards to the door, her ladyship perseveringly pressing him in front. So eager had been the attack on him, that he had not waited to give his order about the post-chaise, but made his way at once towards the hall.

'Now, do'ee take it, do'ee,' pressed Lady Scatcherd.

'Utterly out of the question,' said Dr Fillgrave, with great deliberation, as he backed his way into the hall. As he did so, of course he turned round,—and he found himself almost in the arms of Dr Thorne.

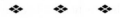

Dr Thorne stepped back three steps and took his hat from his head, having, in the passage from the hall-door to the dining-room, hitherto omitted to do so. It must be borne in mind that he had no conception whatever that Sir Roger had declined to see the physician for whom he had sent; none whatever that that physician was now about to return, feeless, to Barchester.

Dr Thorne and Dr Fillgrave were doubtless well-known enemies. All the world of Barchester, and all that portion of the world of London which is concerned with the lancet and the scalping-knife, were well aware of this: they were continually writing against each other; continually speaking against each other; but yet they had never hitherto come to that positive personal collision which is held to justify a cut direct. They very rarely saw each other; and when they did meet, it was in some casual way in the streets of Barchester or elsewhere, and on such occasions their habit had been to bow with very cold propriety.

On the present occasion, Dr Thorne of course felt that Dr Fillgrave had the whip-hand of him; and, with a sort of manly feeling on such a point, he conceived it to be most compatible with his own dignity to show, under such circumstances, more than his usual courtesy—something, perhaps, amounting almost to cordiality. He had been supplanted, *quoad* (as) doctor, in the house of this rich, eccentric, railway baronet, and he would show that he bore no malice on that account.

So he smiled blandly as he took off his hat, and in a civil speech he expressed a hope that Dr Fillgrave had not found his patient to be in any very unfavourable state.

Here was an aggravation to the already lacerated feelings of the injured man. He had been brought thither to be scoffed and scorned at, that he might be a laughing-stock to his enemies, and food for mirth to the vile-minded. He swelled with noble anger till he would have burst, had it not been for the opportune padding of his frock-coat.

'Sir, said he; 'sir:' and he could hardly get his lips open to give vent to the tumult of his heart. Perhaps he was not wrong; for it may be that his lips were more eloquent than would have been his words.

'What's the matter?' said Dr Thorne, opening his eyes wide, and addressing Lady Scatcherd over the head and across the hairs of the irritated man below him. 'What on earth is the matter? Is anything wrong with Sir Roger?'

'Oh, laws, doctor!' said her ladyship. 'Oh, laws; I'm sure it ain't my fault. Here's Dr Fillgrave in a taking, and I'm quite ready to pay him,—quite. If a man gets paid, what more can he want?' And she again held out the five-pound note over Dr Fillgrave's head.

What more, indeed, Lady Scatcherd, can any of us want, if only we could keep our tempers and feelings a little in abeyance? Dr Fillgrave, however, could not so keep his; and, therefore, he did want something more, though at the present moment he could have hardly said what.

Lady Scatcherd's courage was somewhat resuscitated by the presence of her ancient trusty ally; and moreover, she began to conceive that the little man before her was unreasonable beyond all conscience in his anger, seeing that that for which he was ready to work had been offered to him without any work at all.

'Madam,' said he, again turning round at Lady Scatcherd, 'I was never before treated in such a way in any house in Barsetshire—never—never.'

'Good heavens, Dr Fillgrave!' said he of Greshamsbury, 'what is the matter?'

'I'll let you know what is the matter, sir,' said he, turning round again as quickly as before. 'I'll let you know what is the matter. I'll publish this, sir, to the medical world;' and as he shrieked out the words of the threat, he stood on tiptoes and brandished his eye-glasses up almost into his enemy's face.

'Don't be angry with Dr Thorne,' said Lady Scatcherd. 'Any ways, you needn't be angry with him. If you must be angry with anybody—'

'I shall be angry with him, madam,' ejaculated Dr Fillgrave, making another sudden demi-pirouette. 'I am angry with him—or, rather, I despise him;' and completing the circle, Dr Fillgrave again brought himself round in full front of his foe.

Dr Thorne raised his eyebrows and looked inquiringly at Lady Scatcherd; but there was a quiet sarcastic motion round his mouth which by no means had the effect of throwing oil on the troubled waters.

'I'll publish the whole of this transaction to the medical world, Dr Thorne—the whole of it; and if that has not the effect of rescuing the people of Greshamsbury out of your hands, then then—then, I don't know what will. Is my carriage—that is, post-chaise there?' and Dr Fillgrave, speaking very loudly, turned majestically to one of the servants.

'What have I done to you, Dr Fillgrave,' said Dr Thorne, now absolutely laughing, 'that you should determine to take my bread out of my mouth? I am not interfering with your patient. I have come here simply with reference to money matters appertaining to Sir Roger.'

'Money matters! Very well—very well; money matters. That is your idea of medical practice! Very well—very well. Is my post-chaise at the door? I'll publish it all to the medical world every word—every word of it, every word of it.'

'Publish what, you unreasonable man?'

'Man! sir; whom do you call a man? I'll let you know whether I'm a man—post-chaise there!'

'Don't 'ee call him names now, doctor; don't 'ee pray don't 'ee,' said Lady Scatcherd.

By this time they had all got somewhat nearer the hall-door; but the Scatcherd retainers were too fond of the row to absent themselves willingly at Dr Fillgrave's bidding, and it did not appear that any one went in search of the post-chaise.

'Man! sir; I'll let you know what it is to speak to me in that style. I think, sir, you hardly know who I am.'

'All that I know of you at present is, that you are my friend Sir Roger's physician, and I cannot conceive what has occurred to make you so angry.' And as he spoke, Dr Thorne looked carefully at him to see whether that pump-discipline had in truth been applied. There were no signs whatever that cold water had been thrown upon Dr Fillgrave.

'My post-chaise—is my post-chaise there? The medical world shall know all; you may be sure, sir, the medical world shall know it all;' and thus, ordering his post-chaise, and threatening Dr Thorne with the medical world, Dr Fillgrave made his way to the door.

But the moment he put on his hat he resumed. 'No, madam,' said he. 'No; it is quite out of the question: such an affair is not to be arranged by such means. I'll publish it all to the medical world—post-chaise there!' and then, using all his force, he flung as far as he could into the hall a light bit of paper. It fell at Dr Thorne's feet, who, raising it, found that it was a five-pound note.

'I put it into his hat just while he was in his tantrum,' said Lady Scatcherd. 'And I thought that perhaps he would not find it till he got to Barchester. Well, I wish he'd been paid, certainly, although Sir Roger wouldn't see him;' and in this manner Dr Thorne got some glimpse of understanding into the cause of the great offence.

'I wonder whether Sir Roger will see *me*,' said he, laughing.

Sir Roger's Appeal to Dr. Thorne

Anthony Trollope

It was not worth the doctor's while to aver that the testiness had all been on the other side, and that he had never lost his good-humour; so he merely smiled, and asked Sir Roger if he could do anything further for him.

'Indeed you can, doctor; and that's why I sent for you,—why I sent for you yesterday. Get out of the room, Winterbones,' he then said, gruffly, as though he were dismissing from his chamber a dirty dog. Winterbones, not a whit offended, again hid his cup under his coat-tail and vanished.

'Sit down, Thorne, sit down,' said the contractor, speaking quite in a different manner from any that he had yet assumed. 'I know you're in a hurry, but you must give me half an hour. I may be dead before you can give me another; who knows?'

The doctor of course declared that he hoped to have many a half-hour's chat with him for many a year to come.

'Well, that's as may be. You must stop now, at any rate. You can make the cob pay for it, you know.'

The doctor took a chair and sat down. Thus entreated to stop, he had hardly any alternative but to do so.

'It wasn't because I'm ill that I sent for you, or rather let her ladyship send for you. Lord bless you, Thorne; do you think I don't know

From Anthony Trollope, *Dr. Thorne* (New York: Penguin, 1991), pp. 124–127, 128–129.

what it is that makes me like this? When I see that poor wretch, Winterbones, killing himself with gin, do you think I don't know what's coming to myself as well as him?'

'Why do you take it then? Why do you do it? Your life is not like his. Oh, Scatcherd! Scatcherd!' and the doctor prepared to pour out the flood of his eloquence in beseeching this singular man to abstain from his well-known poison.

'Is that all you know of human nature, doctor? Abstain. Can you abstain from breathing, and live like a fish does under water?'

'But Nature has not ordered you to drink, Scatcherd.'

'Habit is second nature, man; and a stronger nature than the first. And why should I not drink? What else has the world given me for all that I have done for it? What other resource have I? What other gratification?'

'Oh, my God! Have you not unbounded wealth? Can you not do anything you wish? be anything you choose?'

'No,' and the sick man shrieked with an energy that made him audible all through the house. 'I can do nothing that I would choose to do; be nothing that I would wish to be! What can I do? What can I be? What gratification can I have except the brandy bottle? If I go among gentlemen, can I talk to them? If they have anything to say about a railway, they will ask me a question: if they speak to me beyond that, I must be dumb. If I go among my workmen, can they talk to me? No; I am their master, and a stern master. They bob their heads and shake in their shoes when they see me. Where are my friends? Here!' said he, and he dragged a bottle from under his very pillow. 'Where are my amusements? Here!' and he brandished the bottle almost in the doctor's face. 'Where is my one resource, my one gratification, my only comfort after all my tolls? Here, doctor; here, here, here!' and, so saying, he replaced his treasure beneath his pillow.

There was something so horrifying in this, that Dr Thorne shrank back amazed, and was for a moment unable to speak.

'But, Scatcherd,' he said at last; 'surely you would not die for such a passion as that?'

'Die for it? Aye, would I. Live for it while I can live; and die for it when I can live no longer. Die for it! What is that for a man to do? Do not men die for a shilling a day? What is a man the worse for dying? What can I be the worse for dying? A man can die but once, you said just now. I'd die ten times for this.'

'You are speaking now either in madness, or else in folly, to startle me.'

'Folly enough, perhaps, and madness enough, also. Such a life as mine makes a man a fool, and makes him mad, too. What have I about me that I should be afraid to die? I'm worth three hundred thousand pounds; and I'd give it all to be able to go to work tomorrow with a hod and mortar, and have a fellow clap his hand upon my shoulder, and say: "Well, Roger, shall us have that 'ere other half-pint this morning?" I'll tell you what, Thorne, when a man has made three hundred thousand pounds, there's nothing left for him but to die. It's all he's good for then. When money's been made, the next thing is to spend it. Now the man who makes it has not the heart to do that.'

The doctor, of course, in hearing all this, said something of a tendency to comfort and console the mind of his patient. Not that anything he could say would comfort or console the man; but that it was impossible to sit there and hear such fearful truths—for as regarded Scatcherd they were truths—without making some answer.

'This is as good as a play, isn't it, doctor?' said the baronet. 'You didn't know how I could come out like one of those actor fellows. Well, now, come; at last I'll tell you why I have sent for you. Before that last burst of mine I made my will.'

'You had a will made before that.'

'Yes, I had. That will is destroyed. I burnt it with my own hand, so that there should be no mistake about it. In that will I had named two executors, you and Jackson. I was then partner with Jackson in the York and Yeovil Grand Central. I thought a deal of Jackson then. He's not worth a shilling now.'

'Well, I'm exactly in the same category.'

'No, you're not. Jackson is nothing without money; but money'll never make you.'

'No, nor I shan't make money,' said the doctor.

'No, you never will. Nevertheless, there's my other will, there, under that desk there; and I've put you in as sole executor.'

'You must alter that, Scatcherd; you must indeed; with three hundred thousand pounds to be disposed of, the trust is far too much for any one man: besides you must name a younger man; you and I are of the same age, and I may die the first.'

'Now, doctor, doctor, no humbug; let's have no humbug from you. Remember this: if you're not true, you're nothing.'

'Well, but, Scatcherd—'

'Well, but, doctor, there's the will, it's already made. I don't want to consult you about that. You are named as executor, and if you have the heart to refuse the act when I'm dead, why, of course you can do so.'

The doctor was no lawyer, and hardly knew whether he had any means of extricating himself from this position in which his friend was determined to place him.

'You'll have to see that will carried out, Thorne. Now I'll tell you what I have done.'

'You're not going to tell me how you've disposed of your property?'

'Not exactly; at least not all of it. One hundred thousand I've left in legacies, including, you know, what Lady Scatcherd will have.'

'Have you not left the house to Lady Scatcherd?'

'No; what the devil would she do with a house like this? She doesn't know how to live in it now she has got it. I have provided for her; it matters not how. The house and the estate, and the remainder of my money, I have left to Louis Philippe.'

'What! two hundred thousand pounds?' said the doctor.

'And why shouldn't I leave two hundred thousand pounds to my son, even to my eldest son if I had more than one? Does not Mr Gresham leave all his property to his heir? Why should not I make an eldest son as well as Lord de Courcy or the Duke of Omnium? I suppose a railway contractor ought not to be allowed an eldest son by Act of Parliament! Won't my son have a title to keep up? And that's more than the Greshams have among them.'

The doctor explained away what he said as well as he could. He could not explain that what he had really meant was this, that Sir Roger Scatcherd's son was not a man fit to be trusted with the entire control of an enormous fortune.

Sir Roger Scatcherd had but one child; that child which had been born in the days of his early troubles, and had been dismissed from his mother's breast in order that the mother's milk might nourish the young heir of Greshamsbury. The boy had grown up, but had become strong neither in mind nor body. His father had determined to make a gentleman of him, and had sent him to Eton and to Cambridge. But even this receipt, generally as it is recognised, will not make a gentleman. It is hard, indeed, to define what receipt will do so, though people do have in their own minds some certain undefined, but yet tolerably correct ideas on the subject. Be that as it may, two years at Eton, and three terms at Cambridge, did not make a gentleman of Louis Philippe Scatcherd.

Yes; he was christened Louis Philippe, after the King of the French [1773–1850].

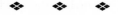

There was nothing royal about Louis Philippe Scatcherd but his name. He had now come to man's estate, and his father, finding the Cambridge receipt to be inefficacious, had sent him abroad to travel with a tutor. The doctor had from time to time heard tidings of this youth; he knew that he had already shown symptoms of his father's vices, but no symptoms of his father's talents; he knew that he had begun life by being dissipated, without being generous; and that at the age of twenty-one he had already suffered from delirium tremens.

It was on this account that he had expressed disapprobation, rather than surprise, when he heard that his father intended to bequeath the bulk of his large fortune to the uncontrolled will of this unfortunate boy.

'I have toiled for my money hard, and I have a right to do as I like with it. What other satisfaction can it give me?'

The doctor assured him that he did not at all mean to dispute this.

'Louis Philippe will do well enough, you'll find,' continued the baronet, understanding what was passing within his companion's breast. 'Let a young fellow sow his wild oats while he is young, and he'll be steady enough when he grows old.'

'But what if he never lives to get through the sowing?' thought the doctor to himself. 'What if that wild-oats operation is carried on in so violent a manner as to leave no strength in the soil for the produce of a more valuable crop?' It was of no use saying this however, so he allowed Scatcherd to continue.

'If I'd had a free fling when I was a youngster, I shouldn't have been so fond of the brandy bottle now. But any way, my son shall be my heir. I've had the gumption to make the money, but I haven't the gumption to spend it. My son, however, shall be able to ruffle it with the best of them. I'll go bail he shall hold his head higher than ever young Gresham will be able to hold his. They are much of the same age, as well I have cause to remember;—and so has her ladyship there.'

Now the fact was, that Sir Roger Scatcherd felt in his heart no special love for young Gresham; but with her ladyship it might almost be a question whether she did not love the youth whom she had nursed almost as well as that other one who was her own proper offspring.

'And will you not put any check on thoughtless expenditure? If you live ten or twenty years, as we hope you may, it will become unnecessary; but in making a will, a man should always remember he may go off suddenly.'

'Especially if he goes to bed with a brandy bottle under his head; eh, doctor? But, mind, that's a medical secret, you know; not a word of that out of the bedroom.'

Dr Thorne could but sigh. What could he say on such a subject to such a man as this?

'Yes, I have put a check upon his expenditure. I will not let his daily bread depend on any man; I have therefore left him five hundred a year at his own disposal, from the day of my death. Let him make what ducks and drakes of that he can.'

'Five hundred a year certainly is not much,' said the doctor.

'No; nor do I want to keep him to that. Let him have whatever he wants if he sets about spending it properly. But the bulk of the property—this estate of Boxall Hill, and the Greshamsbury mortgage, and those other mortgages—I have tied up in this way: they shall be all his at twenty-five; and up to that age it shall be in your power to give him what he wants.'

3

The Cult of Pathology

An Introduction to Selections
from Eugène Sue's Les Mystères de Paris

Eugène Sue (1804–1857), though hardly read and little known today, was in his own time a highly popular writer. His most famous work, *Les Mystères de Paris* (1844), is an extremely long novel with a large cast of characters and a complicated plot. When it was first published in serial form in the magazine *Débats* between June 1842 and October 1843, it was deemed by critics "one of the most important events in French life." It was adapted for the theater in 1844 and again in 1889, but has been translated into English only in an abbreviated, truncated version.

Sue came from a family distinguished in the medical profession for four generations; it comprised fourteen surgeons, five professors, and five members of the French Academy. Although he himself resisted the pressure to become a doctor, he was for a time apprenticed to his father, and spent two further years working in hospitals so that he could draw on intimate, personal experience for the portrayal of the hospital scenes in his novel.

In a lengthy footnote (suppressed in the English translation), appended to the opening of Part 9, chapter 6, Sue makes a kind of apologia for the very negative image he gives of medical practice in hospitals. The illustrious work of his father, grandfather, great-uncle, and great-grandfather, whose name he has the honor to bear, prohibits him, he maintains, from attacking or denigrating the medical profession. This disclaimer serves merely to heighten the gravity of Sue's indictment of the fictional Dr. Griffon as he parades through his ward with his entourage.

The hospital is a place of death, not of healing. Sue evokes its fetid atmosphere, the gloom and sense of doom that engulf all who enter it. As its barred windows suggest, it is like a prison for those who submit to its rules because they have no alternative, no one to care for them at home, and no more strength to sustain themselves. Through his familiarity with hospitals, Sue is able not only to describe the physical environment and the routines but as narrator also to draw us in by invoking readers, making us, as it were, spectators and vicarious participants in the series of dramas being enacted: the death of a nameless patient in the first selection "Death in the Hospital," the extensive examination of Jeanne Duport, and the doctor's pleasure at coming upon a rare disease in a new patient, Claire Fremont (in the third selection, "Rounds").

The central and dominant figure throughout these scenes is that of the doctor in charge, Dr. Griffon in the second selection, "Dr. Griffon." His name itself already implies his predatory nature: a griffin is in ornithology a bird of prey, a type of vulture, and in mythology an animal with the body of a lion and an eagle's head and wings. This doctor devours his patients, and he does so with undisguised relish for the sake of science. He is called a "prince of science," a complimentary designation given to leading nineteenth-century French physicians, but in his case the phrase has a distinctly derisive ring because his behavior, while perhaps princely in its imperiousness, is wholly lacking in nobility. On his rounds he is followed by a throng of assistants and students described as his "scientific cortege." "Cortege," too, is an ambiguous word that can refer in its celebratory sense to the retinue of an eminent personage, yet that carries too a darker resonance through its association with a funeral procession.

As the committed advocate of pathological anatomy, Dr. Griffon appears as the angel of death. He is, as it were, possessed by an obsession with experimentation, using his indigent hospital patients to try out a variety of dangerous drugs, such as iodine, strychnine, arsenic, and phosphorous to combat fever. Even his assistants are astonished at his heedless readiness to take risks. Those therapies that prove successful he will subsequently apply to his paying clientele. From a purely scientific point of view his methods are the proper ones: he conducts controlled experiments by treating one group of patients in a certain innovative way, others by the old method, and leaving a third group untreated so as to be able to compare the outcome. A telling image is applied to Dr. Griffon when he is likened to a general who has won a victory costly in lives. For he is so totally intoxicated by the potential of science and his own power that he is devoid of humanity, compassion, or ethical scruples. He treats his patients with utmost contempt as merely "subjects," that is, material for his research experiments which are justified, in his eyes, because they may further science even if they result in the unnecessary death of some patients. He is unresponsive, indeed blind and deaf to the plight of suffering, frightened creatures. He wholly disregards the shame felt by women, especially young ones, at having to expose their bodies before a male physician and his curious students. Equally brutal is his public exploration of patients' personal lives. When Jeanne talks about her worries over the care of her children, he abruptly interrupts her, refusing to listen to her so as not to disturb his own reflections on the diagnosis. In the face of the patients' distress, Dr. Griffon remains "smiling" and in a jolly mood, pleased at finding such intriguing and challenging cases. A patient who has recently died is just a precious cadaver for dissection to be generously bestowed on a deserving assistant. The fact that the patient is referred to only as a number (number 1) underscores the eradication of any personal individuality, and is an ironic rebuttal of his claim that hospital patients and their doctors form one "large family." In the charity hospital system prevalent through most of the nineteenth century, patients were radically disempowered, having tacitly agreed to hand over their bodies in return for some sort of care, while the physician has the authority, and the right, to exercise unchecked tyranny in the name of science.

Dr. Griffon is shown as so insensitive, vain, and vicious that we are bound to ask whether this image is not exaggerated. Is he a monster, a madman of sadistic savagery, or an example of those "respectable" (Sue's word) doctors whose heads were turned by the exciting possibilities afforded by scientific discoveries? Although Sue maintains in the opening footnote to the hospital chapters of *Les Mystères de Paris* that "this is in no way exaggerated," it seems likely that his own ambivalence toward the medical profession played some part in his presentation of Dr. Griffon. On the other hand, the testimony of extraneous, unprejudiced witnesses, notably visiting foreign physicians, reports disapprovingly of the type of indifference and brutality to patients exhibited by Dr. Griffon. No wonder that hospitals were shunned with horror by all who could possibly avoid submitting to such degradation.

The ruthless methods of this researcher on the cutting edge are in sharp contrast to Dr. Thorne's humane consideration for his patients. In part the difference is one of class: in Trollope's novel the patients are pretty affluent, whereas those in Sue's work are without resources and so have to enter the hospital and become research subjects in order to obtain any measure of care at all. The bodies of those not claimed by relatives for burial are automatically consigned for dissection, a prospect that is a major concern to the dying. The social reality of the charity hospital system is shown in *Les Mystères de Paris* to be conducive to scientific experimentation but immensely detrimental to the health of patients.

Sue's portrayal of a fanatical researcher raises troubling ethical issues. Is it legitimate to use human subjects without their consent for the purpose of research? To what extent do the ends of science justify the means? Trollope's Dr. Thorne was able to do little beyond giving sound advice and comfort; was this old style of practice better for his patients than Dr. Griffon's cult of pathology? Is Dr. Griffon a cautionary figure of science run amuck? Does his extremism cast a shadow over the very idea of scientific experimentation? Can progress be made in medicine without taking risks? What degree of risk to patients is acceptable?

Death in the Hospital

Eugène Sue

Nothing is more lugubrious than the sight of the huge hospital ward at night into which we are taking the reader.

Its great dark walls, punctuated now and then by barred windows as in a prison, are lined by two parallel rows of beds, dimly lit by the funereal light of a lamp suspended from the ceiling.

The atmosphere is so nauseating, so oppressive that recently admitted patients often deteriorate simply in growing used to it; this additional suffering is part of the price that each new arrival has to pay for the sinister stay in hospital. After some time, a certain morbidly dingy color shows that the patient has undergone the initial impact of this noxious environment and has become acclimatized. The air of this enormous ward is heavy and fetid.

The night silence is occasionally interrupted by plaintive groans or deep sighs from those unable to sleep because of their fevers. Then there is quiet, broken only by the regular, monotonous swing of the clock's pendulum marking the very very long hours of those awake in pain. One end of this ward is plunged in almost complete darkness.

Suddenly there is the sound and movement of hurried steps in that area; a door opens and closes several times; a nurse-nun, recognizable by her large white headdress and her black clothing in the light of a lamp

From Eugène Sue, *Les Mystères de Paris* (Paris: Pauvert, 1963), pp. 807–808. Translated by Lilian Furst.

she is carrying, goes to one of the last beds on the right. Some of the patients, abruptly aroused, sit up to see what is happening.

Soon the two wings of the door open. A priest enters carrying a crucifix. The two nuns kneel down. In the dim circle of light surrounding this bed while the rest of the ward remains in darkness, the hospital almoner can be seen bending over this berth of misery, and pronouncing a few words whose muffled sound is lost in the silence of the night.

After a quarter of an hour the priest lifts the end of the sheet and covers the whole bed with it. Then he leaves. One of the kneeling nuns stands up, closes the partition curtains, which creak on their runners, and resumes her prayers next to her fellow nun.

Then silence falls again.

One of the patients has just died.

Dr. Griffon

Eugène Sue

This learned doctor, who had obtained an appointment at this hospital through personal connections, regarded these wards as a forum for experimentation where he might try on the poor the treatments he would later apply to his wealthy patients. On the rich he never risked a new therapeutic method before having several times tried and repeated it *in anima vili* (on commoners), as he called them with that sort of unvarnished viciousness that comes from blind passion and especially from the habit and power of imposing on God's creatures all the capricious experiments and scholarly fantasies of an inventive mind without either fear or supervision.

So, for example, if Dr. Griffon wanted to test the comparative effect of a new and quite dangerous medication in order to be able to ascertain its favorable impact on one organ or another, he would take a certain number of patients, treat one group by the new method, another by the old, and leave others solely to the forces of nature. Afterwards he would count how many had survived. These terrible experiments were, truth to tell, sacrifices on the altar of science.

Dr. Griffon never even thought about it. In the eyes of this prince of science, as the modern designation goes, the patients in his hospital were no more than materials for study and experimentation. And since,

From Eugène Sue, *Les Mystères de Paris* (Paris: Pauvert, 1963), pp. 805–806, 807, 814. Translated by Lilian Furst.

after all, this research sometimes produced a useful fact or a scientific discovery, Dr. Griffon was as naively satisfied and triumphant as a general after a victory that had cost many lives.

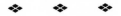

He went on without pity making his patients swallow iodine, stychnine, or arsenic to the extreme limits of *physiological tolerance*, or, to put it plainly, to the extinction of life.

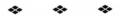

Once the doors of Dr. Griffon's wards were shut behind patients, they belonged body and soul to science. No friendly or impartial ear could hear their lamentations. They were told bluntly that, having been admitted to the hospital as charity cases, they formed thenceforth a part of the doctor's experimental domain. The patient and the disease were to serve as subjects for study, observation, analysis, or the instruction of the young students who assiduously followed Dr. Griffon on his rounds.

The patient had to respond to interrogations that were often most grievous and painful, and were not conducted in private with the physician, as in confession with a priest who has the right to know everything. No, the patients had to reply in a loud voice in front of an avidly curious crowd.

In this pandemonium of science, young and old men, girls and women were obliged to shed any feeling of modesty or shame, to reveal the most intimate details, to submit to the most painful substantive investigations before a numerous audience, and nearly always these cruel practices aggravated their disease.

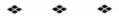

The clock struck seven-thirty.

"Let's go, gentlemen," said Dr. Griffon, and began his rounds with a large following.

When he got to the first bed on the right side, where the partition curtains were drawn, the sister told the doctor:

"Sir, number 1 died at 4.30 A.M."

"As late as that? I'm surprised. Yesterday morning I didn't think she would last out the day. Has the body been claimed?"

"No, sir."

"So much the better; it's a beautiful specimen for autopsy; I'll make someone happy." Then, turning to one of the students following him: "My dear Dunoyer, you've been wanting a cadaver for a long time, you're at the top of the list, this one goes to you."

"Oh! sir, how kind you are!"

"I'd like to be able to reward your zeal more often, my dear friend; but put your mark on this specimen, take possession of it . . . there are so many fellows after the quarry." And the doctor moved on.

With the help of a scalpel the student very delicately inscribed an F and a D [for his name, François Denoyer] on the dead actress's arm so as to take possession, as the doctor put it.

Rounds

Eugène Sue

After quickly visiting several patients who offered nothing strange or interesting, Dr. Griffon came to Jeanne Duport.

Seeing this bustling crowd, jostling around her bed, eager to look and to know, to find out and to learn, the poor woman was seized by trembling fear and shame, and wrapped herself tightly in her bedclothes.

Dr. Griffon's stern, contemplative face, his penetrating gaze, his brow as always furrowed by his habitual reflectiveness, his brusque, brief, impatient words further increased Jeanne's fright.

"A new subject!" said the doctor, glancing at the admission sheet on which was entered the new patient's type of illness. Then he threw a long, searching look at Jeanne.

A deep silence ensued during which the assistants, imitating the prince of science, stared at the patient with curiosity. She, for her part, did not take her eyes off the doctor at whom she looked with anguish; she wanted as far as possible to avoid the painful feelings aroused in her by all these eyes fixed on her.

After several minutes of scrutiny the doctor noticed something abnormal in the yellowish tinge of the patient's eyeballs. He came closer to her, and silently examined the whites of her eyes by pushing the lid down with his finger tip. Then several students, in response to a kind of unspoken

From Eugène Sue, *Les Mystères de Paris* (Paris: Pauvert, 1963), pp. 815–819. Translated by Lilian Furst.

invitation from their professor, came forward one by one to look at Jeanne's eyes.

Next, the doctor proceeded to this interrogation:

"Your name?"

"Jeanne Duport," murmured the patient, more and more scared.

"Your age?"

"Thirty-six and a half."

"Louder. Birthplace?"

"Paris."

"Occupation?"

"Fringe maker."

"Are you married?"

"Alas, yes, sir!" Jeanne replied with a great sigh.

"For how long?"

"Eighteen years."

"Do you have children?"

Here, instead of answering, the poor mother gave way to the tears she had so long held back.

"You are not to cry but to answer. Do you have children?"

"Yes, sir, two small boys, and a sixteen-year-old daughter."

Several questions were put at this point that cannot possibly be repeated. Jeanne managed to satisfy the doctor only in stammers and after severe reprimands from him. The poor woman was dying of shame at being made to answer such queries out loud and before such a large audience.

Totally absorbed in his scientific concerns, without any heed whatsoever of Jeanne's excrutiating mortification, the doctor went on:

"How long have you been sick?"

"Four days, sir," said Jeanne, wiping away her tears.

"Tell me how your sickness began."

"Sir, . . . it's . . . there are so many people here. I dare not . . ."

"Come off it! Don't you know the way things work, my dear friend," the doctor said impatiently. "Do you want me to bring a confessional here? Speak out . . . and hurry up."

"By God, sir, these are family matters."

"Don't worry about that, we are like a family here, a large family," added the prince of science, who was very cheerful that day. "Come on, get on with it."

More and more intimidated, stammering and hesitant at each word, Jeanne said: "Sir, I had had a quarrel with my husband . . . about my children, I mean, about my daughter . . . he wanted to take her away— But, you see, sir, I didn't want that because of a bad woman he lives with who would be a bad example to my daughter; then my husband, who was drunk . . . oh, sir, . . . if he hadn't been, . . . he wouldn't have done it . . . he pushed me really hard . . . I fell, and a little later began to vomit blood."

"So that's it, your husband pushed you and you fell—that's a fine tale . . . he certainly did more than just push you . . . he must have hit you hard in the stomach, and a good many times . . . perhaps he even trampled on you . . . Come on, answer, tell the truth."

"Oh, sir, I assure you he was drunk . . . or else he wouldn't have been so nasty."

"Nice or nasty, drunk or not, it doesn't matter, my good woman; I'm not a trial judge; my aim is merely to establish a fact precisely: you were thrown down and violently trampled on, weren't you?"

"Alas! yes, sir," said Jeanne, breaking into tears, "and yet I never gave him cause for complaint . . . I work as hard as I can and I . . ."

"The epigastrium must be painful, you must feel a terrific burning there?" the doctor interrupted Jeanne, "you must be experiencing malaise, lassitude, nausea?"

"Yes, sir . . . I came here only out of dire need when my strength wholly failed me; otherwise I wouldn't have left the children, about whom I am so worried . . . they have just me . . . And Catherine . . . oh! I am most anxious about her, sir, . . . if you knew . . ."

"Your tongue!" said Dr. Griffon, again interrupting the patient.

This order struck Jeanne, who had thought to arouse the doctor's pity, as so strange that at first she did not respond and looked at him in astonishment.

"Let's see that tongue that you use so well," said the doctor, smiling; then with his finger tip he pressed down Jeanne's lower jaw. After making his students one after the other touch and examine the subject's tongue in order to define its color and dryness, the doctor meditated for a moment. Overcoming her fear, Jeanne cried out in a trembling voice:

"Sir, I'll tell you everything . . . some neighbors, as poor as I, were willing to look after the children, but only for a week . . . That's already a long time. After that I must get home myself. So I beg you, for the love of God, to cure me as quickly as possible . . . or more or less . . . at least so that I can get up and work, I have only a week . . . because . . ."

"Discolored face, complete prostration, yet her pulse is quite strong and regular," the doctor said imperturbably, pointing to Jeanne. "Gentlemen, take a good look: the caving in, the burning in the epigastrium: all the symptoms certainly denote *hematomosis*, complicated by hepatitis, caused by domestic troubles, indicated by the yellowish tinge of the eyeballs; the subject has received violent blows to the epigastrium and the abdomen; the vomiting of blood is definitely caused by some organic lesion of certain viscera. In this connection I draw your attention to a very, indeed extremely interesting point: the postmortem findings of those who have died of the affliction from which this subject is suffering show extraordinary variations. Often the illness is very acute and grave, carrying the patient off within a few days, yet no trace of it can be found at autopsy; in other cases, the spleen, the liver, the pancreas show more or less deep lesions. Probably the subject we have here has sustained some such lesions; we are, therefore, going to try to ascertain this ourselves, and you too will do so by a careful examination of the patient."

And with a rapid movement Dr. Griffon threw the covers to the foot of the bed, exposing Jeanne in entirety.

We recoil from describing the kind of grievous struggle this unfortunate woman underwent, sobbing, beside herself with shame, imploring the doctor and his audience.

But at the threat: "You will be thrown out of this hospital if you do not submit to its established practices," a menace so crushing to those for whom the hospital is the sole and last resort, Jeanne submitted to a public examination that lasted a long, a very long time. Dr. Griffon analyzed and explained each symptom, and the most studious of his assistants then wanted to link the practical to the theoretical, and to assess for themselves the subject's physical condition.

As a result of this cruel handling Jeanne felt such violent emotions that she a suffered a nervous crisis, for which Dr. Griffon wrote a further prescription.

The round continued.

Dr. Griffon soon came to the bed of Miss Claire de Fremont . . . With a hospital cloth bonnet on her head, Miss Fremont was languidly leaning on the bolster on her bed; despite the ravages of disease, traces of a beauty full of distinction were discernible on this candid, sweet face.

After a night of acute pain, the poor child had lapsed into a sort of febrile slumber, and when the doctor and his scientific cortege had come into the room, the noise of rounds had not awoken her.

"A new subject, gentlemen!" said the prince of science, glancing at the admission sheet handed to him by a student. "Sickness: slow nerve fever . . . Wonderful!" cried the doctor with an expression of deep satisfaction; "if the resident on duty is not mistaken in his diagnosis, this is a fine windfall. I've been wanting to see a slow nerve fever . . . generally that isn't a disease of the poor. These afflictions almost always follow on serious disturbances in the subject's social position, and naturally, the

higher the position, the more serious the disturbance. It is also one of
the most remarkable afflictions on account of its characteristic manifes-
tations. It goes right back to antiquity, the writings of Hippocrates are
quite specific and straightforward in this instance: this fever, as I said, is
nearly always caused by violent grief. Grief, of course, is as old as the
world. However, curiously, before the eighteenth century no one had
given an exact description of this malady. It's Huxham, who brought so
much honor to medicine at that time, it's Huxham, as I say, who first
wrote a monograph on nerve fever, a monograph which has become a
classic . . . and yet it's a disease with a long lineage," added the doctor,
smiling. "Yes, it belongs to that great, ancient, and illustrious family
febris, fever, whose origins are lost in the mists of time. But let us not
rejoice too much, let's see if we really have the good fortune to possess
an example of this rare affliction. This would be doubly desirable because
I have for very long wanted to try out the internal use of phosphorous. . . . Yes, gentlemen," the doctor resumed, hearing a stir of curiosity
in his audience, "yes, gentlemen, phosphorous, it's an extremely strange
and bold experiment I want to try! but *audaces fortuna juvat* (fortune
helps the audacious), and the opportunity is excellent. We will first see
whether the subject will exhibit on all parts of her body, and especially
on her chest, that miliary eruption which is, according to Huxham, so
characteristic a symptom. By palpitating the subject you will yourselves
ascertain that rugiosity that follows on the eruption. But let's not count
our chickens before they are hatched," added the prince of science, who
was in a decidedly jolly mood.

He gently shook Miss Fremont by the shoulder to awake her. The
young girl trembled and opened her big eyes hollowed out by illness.
Imagine her bewilderment, her horror.

While a crowd of men surrounded her bed and devoured her with
their eyes, she felt the doctor's hand remove the bedclothes and slip his
hand into her bed in order to take hers to feel her pulse.

Gathering all her strength into a cry of anguish and terror, Miss
Fremont screamed: "Mother! . . . help! . . . mother!"

4

Blood-Letting and Septic Surgery

An Introduction to Selections from
Gustave Flaubert's Madame Bovary

Gustave Flaubert (1821–1880) is unquestionably one of the very greatest French novelists of all time, and his *Madame Bovary* (1857) an acknowledged masterpiece of world literature.

Flaubert himself came from an eminent medical family; his father was for twenty-five years chief of the hospital in Rouen, the main city in the province, Normandy, where *Madame Bovary* takes place, and where his brother, too, was a leading doctor. Flaubert took special care to assure the accuracy of the details about the surgery Charles Bovary, Emma's husband, performs by reading up on it in medical textbooks.

Charles is not a fully qualified physician but an *officier de santé* (health officer), a much lower rank corresponding to the British "surgeon" of the time or to today's physician's assistant. And even at this level he has had much difficulty in passing the examinations, failing at his first attempt. The difference in training and prerogatives between physicians and health officers was considerable. Candidates for the doctorate in mid-nineteenth-century France had to spend four years at a medical school, pass five demanding examinations, and compose and defend a dissertation in Latin. Health officers, on the other hand, were required to do only three years of schooling and an undemanding oral examination, or alternatively a six-year apprenticeship. With the advances in medicine in the latter half of the century, heated debates took place about the dangers to the public from scantily trained health officers. In *Madame Bovary* Dr. Canivet laments the "disrepute" brought to a "sacred calling" by health officers (see the fourth selection, "Surgery"). Yet despite their relative ignorance, health officers were deemed necessary to provide some health care for the rural peasant population. Efforts to abolish this class of practitioners, begun in 1847, finally succeeded in 1892. Meanwhile the proportion of health officers in France dropped from 40 percent of medical personnel in mid-century to a mere 10 percent by the 1890s.

Health officers were stringently restricted in what they were allowed to do. They could practice only in the state in which they were licensed so that the Bovarys could move from one place to another in Normandy but no further. Health officers were permitted to deal solely with mild, straightforward cases. Thus Charles remains fully within his rights in attending to Rouault's broken leg (described in the first selection, "A Broken Leg"); he recognizes it as a simple fracture that will heal itself in time with rest, and is quite ingenious in improvising a splint and bandages out of materials available on the farm. He plays the role of physician by uttering the words of comfort he thinks appropriate to a doctor and repeating gestures and phrases used by his teachers. In accordance with the custom of the time, Charles is invited to partake of refreshments so that the visit has a social as well as a medical dimension. In attending to Rouault's leg, Charles gets to meet Emma and to become aware of her attractiveness. His success in mending the leg (by leaving it to mend itself!) establishes his reputation among the peasants. Dimly conscious of his own limitations, Charles is extremely cautious, prescribing mainly soothing medications.

Charles is well liked by his peasant clientele (see the second selection, "Settling into Practice") because he is good-natured and prudent in his treatments, sticking to the standard remedies of his day such as bleedings and emetics. His solid moral character, his modesty, even his very blandness endear him to his naive patients, eliciting their trust. The insinuation is that he is not far above their level intellectually. Unlike Trollope's Dr. Thorne (chapter 2) or George Eliot's Lydgate in *Middlemarch* (chapter 5), Charles is not at odds with the social reality in which he works, but this happy consonance stems from a common mediocrity. Although the initial glimpses of Charles's professional activity present a rather favorable image, readers are from the outset also made aware of his innate shortcomings: his knowledge of and interest in medicine are quite superficial, he is by nature inclined to timidity, and his primary method to achieve success is to do as little as possible. This less complimentary view of

Charles is obliquely conveyed to readers by means of the persistent authorial satire and irony. For instance, we are told that he subscribes to a new medical journal *"in order to keep up to date,"*—and promptly falls asleep over it (see the second selection, "Settling into Practice"). The italicization of that phrase denotes a citation of Charles's words. This literary technique of indirect speech recurs throughout the novel, often serving as a vehicle for irony. In the case of Charles, for example, it brings out the discrepancy between his self-image as a healer and the dismal reality. A similar message is contained in the information that he acquires a medical reference book, whose pages remain uncut, unused. So Charles's medical competence is indirectly thrown into question from the very beginning of *Madame Bovary*. Not in a position to distinguish good from bad advice or treatment, his patients mistake his passivity for wisdom, as indeed it is, given his ignorance. So long as he refrains from doing anything beyond pulling a tooth, putting a splint on a broken leg, or prescribing a palliative balm, Charles gets along well enough.

But as soon as he embarks on a more active course, he gets into difficulties, even within the boundaries imposed on health officers. Among the "surgical" procedures sanctioned at this level was blood-letting, a popular therapy at the time for all manner of afflictions. It could be performed either by cutting a vein open, as Charles does, or by applying leeches, which had been imported into France by the million annually earlier in the century, but which, by mid-century, were being superseded by the method of opening a vein (described in "A Blood-Letting," the third selection). In this episode the local squire brings his servant to Charles's home to be bled, thus illustrating the convention that health officers treat the lower classes. The efficacy of blood-letting is dubious in this case since the patient complains of feeling *"ants all over his body,"* suggesting perhaps a neurological or a dermatological disease, or quite likely alcoholism. The unscientific nature of Charles's practice is implied in the adjacency of his office to the kitchen so that the smells of cooking waft into the office while the sounds of coughing and the recital of maladies can be heard in the kitchen. When the pharmacist's apprentice, Justin, who is assisting Charles, faints at the sight of blood, Charles calls in his wife who loosens Justin's clothes and rubs vinegar onto his temples. Just as the office and the kitchen are next to each other, so traditional domestic medicine is closely related to the kind of medicine practiced by health officers, and often domestic remedies are more effective. As Charles struggles to maintain control, the situation has a comic dimension; yet it also has darker implications in revealing his clumsiness in mismanaging even a very commonplace procedure.

Charles's ineptitude in the minor treatment of the bleeding prepares for the central medical fiasco in *Madame Bovary*, the operation (see the fourth selection, "Surgery") on the clubfoot of the groom, Hippolyte. Charles is here clearly transgressing what he is legally authorized to do. Health officers were permitted to give emergency first aid such as ligaturing a major artery to stem bleeding after an accident, but elective surgeries for conditions like harelip, cataract, or clubfoot were categorically forbidden. Deformities like clubfeet were not uncommon in the French countryside as a result of inbreeding through generations of intermarriage among villagers. The surgical treatment of clubfoot was popularized in the press after the publication in 1839 of Dr. Vincent Duval's book, *Traité pratique du pied-bot* (Practical Treatise on Clubfoot). Various instruments and contraptions were invented to repair such defects; however, the solution to the problem of postoperative infection lagged behind purely mechanical skills. Only in the 1860s did Joseph Lister begin to apply carbolic and phenic acid to wounds to prevent putrefaction.

Wary and unenterprising as he is, Charles does not embark on this venture of his own accord. But he is a weak character so that he lets himself be talked into attempting something far beyond his abilities by the sustained persuasion of Homais, the town's pharmacist, who is backed by Emma, Charles's wife. Homais, who has great pretensions to being an enlightened man of science, has read about the innovative surgery in the newspapers. This detail shows the haphazard and shallow way in which information about medical advances was disseminated. Neither Homais nor Emma is motivated by humanitarian considerations for the patient. It is, Homais argues in his overblown rhetoric, in the service of progress and patriotism to keep up with new developments in medicine. He enumerates the hypothetical benefits to the patient and the advantages to the community without a thought to the potential risks involved. Emma is readily convinced; bored with her life and disappointed in Charles, she longs for excitement. Together they prevail upon Charles that this is a sure means to acquire fame and fortune for the town as well as for himself. After some hesitation, Hippolyte, too, is talked into agreeing to the surgery through appeals to his vanity, especially the prospect of enhancing his attractiveness to women.

The procedure itself proves surprisingly easy and uneventful. Flaubert describes with dramatic gusto how the amateur surgeons imitate the experts by aping merely the external trappings such as piles of lint, bandages, and suturing threads. But while an improvised splint sufficed for a simple fracture, the cumbersome contraption used by Charles and assembled with the help of the local carpenter and locksmith, fills the reader with foreboding. Similarly, the muddled references to technical terms from the anatomy textbooks that Charles studies emphasize his confusion; he really has no idea what he is doing. The sense of drama is heightened by the comparison of Charles to such illustrious past practitioners of surgery as Ambroise Paré, Celsus, Dupruyten, and Gensoul. To place Charles in this context is both to make fun of him and to underscore the ludicrous disparity between the achievements of these eminent surgeons and Charles's dismal botching. The speedy, almost abrupt ending to the procedure comes as a calculated anticlimax after the lengthy preparatory build-up.

Five days later infection and gangrene set in. Before antispesis one surgical case in every two-and-a-half resulted in death, and amputations, often also followed by death, were frequent. Neither Charles nor Homais has the slightest inkling of this hazard. In their ignorance they foolishly and stubbornly persist in torturing the patient with their contraption. The unsavoriness of the situation is vividly brought out by the concrete details: the dirty pillows, the swarms of flies, and soon the stench of the gangrenous wound. The seriousness of Hippolyte's condition is, significantly, recognized by his lay caregiver, Madame Lefrançois, rather than by his medical attendants. She also shows better sense than they in resorting to the domestic remedy of feeding him nourishing food in place of the prescribed diet. She supports him psychologically but, like the peasants who drop in on market days, she is skeptical of avant-garde medicine.

When the catastrophic outcome becomes manifest, a fully qualified physician is called from the neighboring town; he immediately amputates the leg without any anesthesia. General anesthesia had been successfully demonstrated in Boston in 1846, and reported in the *Boston Medical and Surgical Journal*, but because of the slow spread of medical advances in those days, word had obviously not reached the depths of the French provinces. Dr. Canivet does not bother to conceal his contempt for Charles, nor does he show any concern for the patient. Though a graduated doctor, he, too, is the object of satire and irony: the care of his horse takes priority over that of the patient, and his confident self-assurance masks a brutal indifference; it is all the same to him whether he is cutting up a "Christian or a chicken." That striking phrase is an indirect indictment of his utter callousness, which he likes to pass off as the virtue of hardiness. Homais, likewise, comes off badly in this crisis, betraying Charles for the sake of his business interests and lacking the fortitude to assist in the amputation. The kindliest among the medical personnel is ultimately the bungling Charles; distraught at the damage he has wrought, he goes on wondering where he went wrong without ever understanding what happened. He endeavors to make amends to Hippolyte by buying him a wooden leg, and for the rest of the novel, in another brilliantly tragi-comic detail, its clippity-clopp sound is a reiterated reminder of Charles's professional inadequacy and stupidity.

Madame Bovary reveals how primitive medicine continued to be in remote rural areas even as momentous advances were being made in the major research centers. Its action is contemporaneous with that of Sue's *Les Mystères de Paris* (chapter 3); the contrast between Dr. Griffon's cult of the scientific approach and Charles Bovary's amateurishness indicates the vast spectrum of medical practice found in the same country and at the same period. Another ironic contrast is that between the willingness of such ignoramuses as the pharmacist and the health officer to experiment with new procedures and the qualified physician's adamant and quite irrational skepticism about "Parisian inventions." The fitful transmission of medical discoveries is illustrated by the reliance on chance newspaper reports, which have brought word of the new French surgery on clubfeet but not of the American discovery of anesthesia.

Flaubert's novel drastically undermines the image of nineteenth-century medicine as a triumphant march of progress. More damaging even than backwardness is the misapplication of valid advances in the hands of those ill prepared to implement them. Are Homais and Charles more of a menace than a help to their patients? How does Charles compare to Trollope's Dr. Thorne (chapter 2) who sticks to the old style of practice? Is the potential for harm by innovations outweighed by the hopes for benefit? That is the crucial question that Homais and Charles never address, but that continues to be an important issue in our day too.

A Broken Leg (Part 1, chapter 2)

Gustave Flaubert

Charles went up to the second floor to see the patient. He found him in bed, perspiring under the bedclothes, and having chucked away his cotton nightcap. He was a small, stout man of about fifty with a fair skin, blue eyes, balding at the front, and wearing earrings. On a chair at his side was a large bottle of brandy to raise his spirits. But as soon as he saw the doctor, his courage left him, and instead of swearing as he had done for the past twelve hours, he began to moan feebly.

It was a simple fracture without any kind of complication. Charles could not have wished for anything easier. Then, recalling his teachers' bedside manners toward the injured, he began to comfort his patient with all sorts of consoling phrases, surgical caresses which are like oil for greasing the skids to the scalpel. So as to make splints, a bundle of slats was brought from the shed. Charles chose one, cut it into pieces, and polished them with a shard from a broken pane while the servant tore up sheets to serve as bandages, and Miss Emma tried to sew some pads. As it took her a long time to find her sewing basket, her father became impatient; in sewing she pricked her fingers which she then put into her mouth to suck.

Charles was surprised at the whiteness of her nails. They were so shiny, tapered, more polished than the ivories of Dieppe, and shaped like

From Gustave Flaubert, *Madame Bovary* (Paris: Garnier, 1947), pp. 15–16. Translated by Lilian Furst.

almonds. But her hand was not beautiful, not pale enough perhaps, and a little dry at the knuckles; it was also too long and devoid of gentle softness in its outline. What was most beautiful about her was her eyes; although they were brown, they looked black because of the lashes, and her look came at you directly with an intrepid candor.

Once the dressing had been done, the doctor was invited by Mr. Rouault himself to *partake of some refreshment* before leaving.

Settling into Practice
(Part 1, chapter 9)

Gustave Flaubert

He was well, and he looked well; his reputation was firmly established. The country folks liked him because he was not pretentious. He fondled their children, never drank in bars, and altogether inspired confidence through his upright way of life. He enjoyed especial success with catarrhs and chest diseases. Terribly afraid of killing his patients, Charles in fact prescribed hardly anything other than soothing potions, an occasional emetic, foot baths, or leeches. It was not that he was afraid of surgery; he bled people copiously as if they were horses, and for pulling teeth he had *the devil of a grip.*

Also, *in order to keep up to date,* he took out a subscription to the *Medical Hive*, a new journal for which he had received a prospectus. He browsed a little in it after dinner, but the warmth of the apartment together with the business of digestion made him fall asleep within five minutes; he would stay there, his chin in his hands, and his hair spread like a mane right to the base of the lamp.

From Gustave Flaubert, *Madame Bovary* (Paris: Garnier, 1947), p. 65. Translated by Lilian Furst.

A Blood-Letting (Part 2, chapter 7)

Gustave Flaubert

Emma was sitting with her elbows on the window sill (she sat there often; in the provinces the window fulfills the function of theaters and walks), and amusing herself by watching the throng of yokels when she noticed a gentleman wearing a green velvet coat. He had yellow gloves on, although there were heavy gaiters on his legs; he was proceeding toward the doctor's house, followed by a peasant whose head was bowed and who looked distracted.

"Can I see the doctor?" he asked Justin [the pharmacist's apprentice] who was chatting at the door with the maid, Felicity.

And, taking him for the servant of the house:

"Tell him that Mr. Rodolphe Boulanger of La Huchette is here."

It was not out of territorial pride that the newcomer had added the place to his own name but in order better to establish his identity. La Huchette was a property near Yonville; he had just acquired its manor together with two farms that he looked after himself more or less as a hobby. He was a bachelor, reputed to have *at least fifteen thousand francs a year.*

Charles entered the room. Mr. Boulanger introduced his employee who wanted to be bled because he had the sensation of *ants swarming along his body.*

From Gustave Flaubert, *Madame Bovary* (Paris: Garnier, 1947), pp. 134–136. Translated by Lilian Furst.

"It will clean me out," he insisted in the face of all persuasion to the contrary.

So Bovary began to bring a bandage and a basin, and asked Justin to hold it. Then, turning to the villager, who was already pale:

"Don't be afraid, my good man."

"No, not at all," the other replied, "go ahead!"

And, with a show of bravado, he held out his sturdy arm. At the cut of the lancet the blood spurted out so far as to splash the mirror.

"Bring the basin nearer," Charles shouted.

"Wow!" said the peasant, "it's gushing out like a little fountain! What red blood I have! That must be a good sign, don't you think?"

"Sometimes," replied the health officer, "patients feel nothing at the beginning, then they faint, especially big husky fellows like this one."

At these words the peasant dropped the surgical case he was fingering. A jolt of his shoulders made the back of the chair creak. His hat fell off.

"I'm not surprised," said Bovary, pressing his finger to the vein.

The basin began to tremble in Justin's hands; his knees buckled, he turned pale.

"My wife! My wife!" Charles called out.

In a jiffy she came downstairs.

"Vinegar!" he shouted, "Oh, my God, two of them at once!"

And he was so upset that he had trouble holding the compress.

"It's no big deal," said Mr. Boulanger calmly while he supported Justin in his arms.

And he sat him on the table, propping his back to the wall.

Madame Bovary began to loosen his tie. There was a knot on the strings of his shirt; she spent several minutes untying it; then she poured some vinegar onto her fine handkerchief, moistened his temples with small strokes, and blew on the spot, delicately.

The farmhand came to; but Justin's faint persisted; the pupils of his eyes faded into his white eyeballs like blue flowers in milk.

"We must hide this from him," said Charles.

Madame Bovary took the basin to put it under the table; . . . Then she went to fetch a jug of water in which she was just dissolving pieces of sugar when the pharmacist arrived on the scene. In the heat of the incident the maid had run to fetch him; seeing his apprentice open his eyes, he heaved a sigh of relief.

Surgery (Part 2, chapter 11)

Gustave Flaubert

He [Homais, the pharmacist] had recently read praise of a new method for curing club feet, and as he was an advocate of progress, he conceived the patriotic idea that Yonville ought to engage in orthopedic sugery in order *to get itself put onto the map*.

"For," he said to Emma, "what's the risk? Let's consider it" (and he enumerated on his fingers the advantages of such an attempt): "almost certain success, relief and beautification for the sufferer, rapidly acquired celebrity for the operator. Why would your husband, for instance, not want to rid poor Hippolyte of the *Golden Lion* of his deformity? Note that he wouldn't fail to tell travelers of his cure, and then" (Homais lowered his voice and looked around) "who would stop him [Homais] from sending a little report about it to a newspaper? And, my word, an article gets around . . . , people talk about it . . . , in the long run it's like the proverbial snowball! Who knows? who knows?"

Bovary could indeed succeed; there was nothing to make Emma believe that he was not skillful, and what satisfaction for her to have persuaded him to take a step that would enhance his reputation and fortune. She so badly wanted to have something more solid to depend on than love.

From Gustave Flaubert, *Madame Bovary* (Paris: Garnier, 1947), pp. 184–187, 189–191, 192–195. Translated by Lilian Furst.

When Charles was solicited by the pharmacist and by her, he let himself be talked into it. He had Dr. Duval's volume sent from Rouen, and every evening, his head between his hands, he steeped himself in reading it.

While he was studying the equine, the varus, and valgus, that is to say various types of orthopedic malformation (or, in simpler terms, the different twisting of the foot, downward, inward, or outward) together with orthopedic interventions (in other words, upward torsion or downward realignment), Homais was exhorting the groom at the inn by means of all sorts of arguments to submit to the surgery.

"You'll hardly feel, perhaps, a slight discomfort; it's a little stick, like a small blood-letting, less than the removal of some corns."

Hippolyte rolled his stupid eyes as he thought it over.

"Anyway," the pharmacist went on, "it's your life, not mine! My concern is purely for humanity! I'd like to see you, my friend, rid of that hideous deformity and the swaying in your lumbar region which, however much you conceal it, must hinder you substantially in carrying out your work."

Then Homais put it to him how much livelier and more active he would feel afterwards, and even made him think that he would be more likely to please women, and the stable boy began to grin bashfully. Then Homais went for his vanity:

"Aren't you a man, for heaven's sake? What would it be like if you had had to serve in the army and fight for your country? . . . Oh, Hippolyte!"

So Homais went away, saying that he did not understand this obstinacy, this blindness, this refusal to benefit by science.

The unfortunate boy gave in because it was like a conspiracy. Binet, who never got involved in other people's affairs, Madame Lefrançois, Artemis, the neighbors, even the mayor, Mr. Tuvache, everyone urged him, preached to him, made him feel ashamed; but what clinched his decision *was that it wouldn't cost him anything.* Bovary even assumed responsibility for providing the equipment for the surgery. This generosity had been Emma's idea, and Charles agreed to it, thinking at the bottom of his heart that his wife was an angel.

With the pharmacist's advice and at the third attempt, he got the carpenter, helped by the locksmith, to construct a sort of box that weighed about eight pounds. In making it, they did not save on iron, wood, tin, leather, screws, or bolts.

However, in order to know which tendon to cut in Hippolyte's case, it was essential to find out first what sort of club foot he had.

His foot formed almost a straight line with the leg, and was also turned inward so that it was an equine type with some admixture of the varus, or maybe a mild varus with a strong measure of the equine. But with this equine, truly as large as a horse's hoof with calloused skin, stiff tendons, huge toes, and black nails like those in a horseshoe, the deformed groom galloped about all day long like a deer. He was seen constantly on the main square leaping among the carriages, thrusting his lame foot forward. That leg even seemed stronger than the other. As a result of long use, it had developed as it were moral qualities of patience and energy; and when Hippolyte had a particularly arduous task to perform, he preferred to support himself on that leg.

Since it was of the equine type, the Achilles tendon had to be cut in preparation for later attacking the anterior tibial muscle so as to get rid of the varus. For the doctor did not dare to risk two operations at one go, and even so he already trembled with fear at getting into some important area he did not know.

Not Ambroise Paré applying a ligature directly to an artery for the first time since Celsus fifteen centuries earlier; not Dupruyten opening an abscess through a dense layer of brain tissue; not Gensoul performing the first ablation of the upper maxiliary—none of these for sure had as pounding a heart, as trembling a hand, or as tense a mood as Mr. Bovary when he approached Hippolyte holding his *tenotome*. And, as in hospitals, on a table at the side there was a pile of lint, waxed suturing threads, lots of bandages, a pyramid of bandages, all the bandages from the pharmacy. It was Mr. Homais who had taken charge of all these preparations from early in the morning onward, as much to dazzle the crowd as to nurture his own illusions. Charles pierced the skin; a sharp cracking was heard. The tendon was cut, the operation done. Hippolyte could not get over his surprise; he bent over Bovary's hands to cover them in kisses.

"Now then, calm down," said the pharmacist, "you will express your gratitude to your benefactor later!"

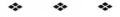

Five days later Madame Lefrançois rushed in, screaming in fright:

"Help! help! he's dying! . . . I don't know what to do!"

Charles rushed to the *Golden Lion*, and the pharmacist who saw him cross the square hatless left his store. He, too, turned up, panting, red, anxious, asking everyone going upstairs:

"What's up with our interesting patient?"

The patient was writhing in such atrocious convulsions that the mechanical contraption in which the leg was encased was banging against the wall with a vehemence fit to break a hole in it.

With great care so as not to disturb the limb's position, the box was removed. A dreadful sight was exposed. The contours of the foot had disappeared under a swelling of such magnitude that the entire skin seemed close to bursting open, and it was covered with bruises caused by the famous contraption. Hippolyte had been complaining of pain; no one had taken any notice; it had to be conceded that he had not been completely wrong, and he was let out of the thing for a few hours. But hardly had the edema subsided a little than the two experts thought it appropriate to put the limb back in the box, fixing it tighter so as to hurry matters up. Eventually, three days later, when Hippolyte could not stand it any longer, they took the contraption off again, and were very surprised at what they saw. A livid tumescence was spreading up the leg with lesions in various spots from which a black liquid was oozing. The enterprise was taking a serious turn for the worse. Hippolyte was beginning to feel discouraged, and Madame Lefrançois moved him into the small room next to the kitchen so that he might at least enjoy some distraction.

But the tax-collector, who took his dinner there every day, objected bitterly to having such a neighbor. So then Hippolyte was carried to the billiard room.

There he was, groaning under the heavy blankets, pale, with a long beard and hollow eyes, from time to time turning his sweaty head on the dirty pillow where flies would land. Madame Bovary came to see him. She brought him linens for his poultices, and consoled and encouraged him. Actually he did not lack company, especially on market days when the peasants came to play billiards, fencing with their cues, smoking, drinking, singing, and braying all around him.

"How are you?" they said, slapping him on the shoulder. "Not too good by the looks of you. But it's not your fault." And they gave him all sorts of advice.

They told him tales of people who had all been cured by remedies other than his; then by way of consolation they added:

"It's because you are too obedient! get up! you are pampering yourself like a king! oh, never mind, old phony! you don't smell good!"

The gangrene was in fact spreading up the leg. It made Bovary himself sick. He kept coming all the time. Hippolyte looked at him with eyes full of terror and stammered sobbing:

"When will I get better! Help me! I am so wretched, so wretched!"

And as he left, the doctor always recommended diet.

"Don't heed him, my boy," urged Madame Lefrançois, "they've already made enough of a martyr of you! You'll get still weaker! Come on, swallow this!"

And she gave him some good broth, a slice of lamb, a bit of bacon, and little glasses of brandy which he hardly dared to raise to his lips.

However, religion did not seem to help him any more than surgery; the unrelentling putrefaction kept on rising from the extremities toward the trunk. Changing the potions and renewing the poultices were to no avail; day by day the tissue rotted more, and finally Charles responded with an affirmative nod when Madame Lefrançois asked him in despair whether she could not have the celebrated Dr. Canivet come from Neufchatel.

A doctor of medicine, about fifty years old, with a good position and great self-assurance, this colleague did not bother to conceal a contemptuous laugh when he saw the leg gangrenous to the knee. Then after declaring bluntly that it had to be amputated, he went over to the pharmacy to castigate those asses who had reduced the poor fellow to such a state. Taking hold of Mr. Homais's coat by the button, he bawled:

"Those Parisian inventions! So much for the ideas of the gentlemen in the capital! It's like the cures for squints, chloroform, and lithotomy, a pack of monstrous practices that the government should ban! But everyone wants to be a wizard, stuffing patients with remedies without worrying about the consequences. Some of us are not so adventurous; we are not scholarly, or fancy swells; we are simply practitioners, healers, who wouldn't dream of operating on someone who is doing just fine! Straighten a club foot? can club feet be straightened? it's like trying, for example, to straighten a hunchback!"

It was painful for Homais to listen to this diatribe, and he hid his unease beneath a courteous smile since he needed to keep well in with Dr. Canivet whose prescriptions were sometimes dispensed as far afield as Yonville; so he did not take up Bovary's defense, indeed he said nothing; foresaking his principles, he sacrificed his dignity in the interests of his business.

This amputation to the thigh by Dr. Canivet created quite a stir in the village! That day everyone got up early, and Main Street, though crowded with people, had a lugubrious air as if an execution were to take place. Hippolyte's illness was discussed at the grocer's; nothing was sold in the shops; and Madame Tuvache, the mayor's wife, did not budge from her window, so impatient was she to see the operator's arrival.

He arrived in his carriage which he drove himself. But since the spring on the right side had over the years come to sag under the weight of his corpulence, the carriage tilted slightly as it moved. On the cushion next to him sat a huge box, covered in red leather; its brass locks gleamed impressively.

When he had swept like a whirlwind through the entrance to the *Golden Lion*, the doctor in a loud order commanded his horse to be unharnessed, then he went into the stable to see that the animal was getting good oats; for when he arrived to see patients, he first took care of his mare and his carriage. Because of this habit it was even said of him: "Oh, Dr. Canivet is an eccentric!" And he was more highly regarded for this unflappable poise. The universe could have fallen apart down to the very last man, and he would not have missed out on a single one of his habits.

Homais appeared on the scene.

"I am counting on you," said the doctor. "Are we ready? Let's go!"

But, blushing, the pharmacist admitted that he was too sensitive to be present at such an operation.

"When you are just a spectator," he said, "the imagination, you know, runs away with you! And, besides, I have such a nervous constitution . . ."

"Nonsense," interrupted Canivet, "you strike me on the contrary as inclined to apoplexy. Anyway, that doesn't surprise me, you pharmacists are constantly cooped up in your kitchens, and that must finally affect your temperament. Look at me, by contrast: every day I get up at four A.M., I shave in cold water (I never feel cold), I don't wear flannel, I don't catch cold, my chest is strong! I live like a stoic philosopher, taking things as they come. That's because I am not squeamish like you; it's all the same to me to cut up a Christian or a chicken. From then on, you'll say, it's a matter of habit . . . , sheer habit . . . !"

Then, without any consideration for Hippolyte, who was sweating under his sheets, these gentlemen engaged in a conversation in which the pharmacist compared the surgeon's composure to a general's; and this comparison pleased Canivet, who proceeded to expostulate in fine terms on the challenges of his art. He regarded it as a sacred calling, although health officers brought it into disrepute. Finally, turning back to the patient, he examined the bandages brought by Homais, the very same ones as had appeared at the operation on the club foot, and asked for someone to hold the limb for him. Lestiboudois was sent for, and Dr.

Canivet rolled up his sleeves, and went into the billiard room while the pharmacist stayed behind with his son, Artemise, and the innkeeper, both of whom were whiter than their aprons; all three kept their ears glued to the door.

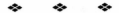

The silence that hung over the village was rent by a harrowing scream.

5

Germs, Drugs, Diagnoses, and Cadavers

An Introduction to Selections from George Eliot's Middlemarch

George Eliot is the pen-name of Mary Ann Evans (1819–80), often considered the leading British nineteenth-century novelist. Her outstanding novel *Middlemarch* derives its name from the prototypical small town in the English provinces that is the scene of the action.

Although *Middlemarch* was published in 1872, its happenings occur some forty years earlier just before the British parliament passed the Reform Bill in May 1832. It not only abolished so-called "rotten" (i.e., corrupt) boroughs and gave votes uniformly to property-owners, but also stimulated a gradual series of further reforms in factory conditions, education, and public health. Passage of the Reform Bill into the Reform Act of Parliament therefore marks an important turning-point in British history. Discussion of the Reform Bill in the months before it was ratified forms the backdrop to the plot of *Middlemarch* so that the novel's overarching theme is reform, social change, and resistance to it, as exemplified in its impact on both individuals and groups. One area of reform prominent throughout *Middlemarch* is that of medical practice. Eliot took great care to become well informed on the beliefs, controversies, and problems in the medical profession. The notebook she kept preparatory to writing the novel has been published as *Quarry to "Middlemarch"*; its entire first half is devoted to medical matters.

Middlemarch's five long-established practitioners are depicted as conservatives who see no need for any change, a stance in which they have the backing of the majority of the town's inhabitants, who are suspicious and afraid of innovations. The clash between the old and the new in medical practice is precipitated by the recent arrival of a young medical man, Lydgate. Although he is properly deferential to individual patients, such as the aristocratic Lady Chettam, whose support he wins, he holds some advanced ideas that he has picked up during his studies in Paris (described in the first selection, "A Conflict of Opinions"). Opinion about Lydgate is sharply divided in the town: its more progressive members, like the gentleman-farmer Brooke and the banker Bulstrode, recognize that "medical knowledge is at a low ebb among us," and would welcome Lydgate's reforms. The opposition, averse to change, is represented by the lawyer Standish, who does not object to the convention of experimentation on charity cases in hospital, but wants himself to be shielded from anything that smacks of novelty. Bulstrode and Standish have long been at loggerheads over the way in which Middlemarch should be run. The short exchange between the two sides near the beginning of the novel rapidly summarizes the dichotomized attitudes toward Lydgate, and reveals how tensions in the town are projected onto him even before he has taken any action at all. So the antagonism to him is partly an irrational extension of already existing divisions.

The conflict between the old and the new first surfaces in the heated debate about the new hospital being planned. Bulstrode, the banker who wields considerable power in the town, recruits Lydgate for this project (see the second selection, "The New Hospital"). The newcomer advocates that part of the hospital should be designated as an isolation area for fevers. This is an issue of immediate concern with the advance through Europe of a cholera epidemic that is threatening to spread to England. But most Middlemarchers see no reason for isolation; they still adhere to the notion current before germ theory (see Introduction) that diseases such as cholera are caused by "miasma," foul air rising from swamps and marshes, not spread by contagion. Lydgate is warned by Bulstrode not to "shrink from incurring a certain amount of jealousy and dislike among your professional brethren by presenting yourself as a reformer." Lydgate's reformist zeal stems from his adherence to "a scientific culture of which country practitioners have usually no more notion than the man in the moon."

What distinguishes Lydgate from the other medical men in Middlemarch? The answer comes largely in the account (see the third selection, "Lydgate's Ideals") of his training and ideals, which depart from the norm in many respects. Lydgate is introduced as the "new surgeon," but the term "surgeon" had then quite a different meaning from what it does nowadays. A nineteenth-century British surgeon held a rather modest rank, although higher than that of a French health officer such as Charles Bovary (chapter 4). The medical profession in Britain in the early nineteenth century was structured according to a definite hierarchy. Physicians, called "Dr.," educated at Oxford or Cambridge, and considered "gentlemen," formed the top category; with their relatively high fees (and, frequently, pretensions) they were mostly patronized by the upper classes. While they received a fine education in the classics so that they could be polished conversationalists, they were given fairly scant training in medicine. At the other end of the spectrum were apothecaries, who were regarded as mere tradesmen because their main function was to sell medications, although they also gave advice, primarily to the lower classes. "Surgeons" were rather precariously situated above apothecaries and below physicians; traditionally trained by apprenticeship, they were supposed to treat only "outward," not internal diseases, which were the physicians' prerogative, and they also dispensed medications. Their more modest fees (and bearing) made them congenial to the emergent middle class. At the time of *Middlemarch* some flexibility was beginning to appear in regard to surgeons who were rising in standing. As a trade guild they had broken away from the Company of Surgeon-Barbers in 1745 to form a separate Company of Surgeons, which became the Royal College of Surgeons with the granting of a charter in 1800. This mid-level of surgeons was on the verge of developing into general (or family) practitioners.

Lydgate works in Middlemarch as changes are just about to begin. He is an outsider, and in many ways an exceptional figure, far above the town's other surgeons, in that he comes from a family with aristocratic connections (like Trollope's Dr. Thorne), and in having undergone extensive further training in London, Edinburgh, and Paris after completing his apprenticeship. Paris was then the site of the most advanced medical research, notably in pathological anatomy, which laid the foundations for the shift from the ancient humoral system to an understanding of disease specificity, i.e., that afflictions can be localized through identification as lesions in one organ or another (see Cadavers section in Introduction). The attraction of the new science was so intense that between 1822 and 1824 courses in normal and pathological anatomy were taught in Paris in English for the many foreign doctors who flocked there for instruction. Lydgate is neatly contextualized in medical history as having been one of those students. In Paris he had become fascinated with the discoveries of the pathologist Bichat, whose work he wants to continue. He intends to engage in research on "primary webs or tissues" (now known as connective tissue) as well as to practice in Middlemarch. He takes as his model Edward Jenner (1749–1823), an English country surgeon like himself, who successfully devised innoculation against small-pox in 1796 through observation of dairy workers with cowpox, a mild form of the disease, on which he based his experiments.

Lydgate's excellent knowledge of medicine at first brings him re-peated success, above all in making the right diagnosis, but also in car-rying out the appropriate treatment as far was feasible in those days. Using the stethoscope he had acquired in Paris, he diagnoses the elderly Casaubon's degenerative heart disease. Drawing on his clinical experi-ence, he recognizes in Fred Vincy "the pink-skinned stage of typhoid fever" which the family's regular attendant, the surgeon Wrench, had dismissed as " 'a minor derangement' " (see the fourth selection, "A Case of Typhoid Fever"). In this incident he is very meticulous about observ-ing the proper "medical etiquette" in meeting with Wrench to discuss the case so as not to be seen as stealing patients from others. Neverthe-less, Lydgate's medical astuteness fuels the opposition to him, partly no doubt owing to jealousy of his success. The disapproval among his peers becomes even more pronounced after his examination of Nancy Nash convinces him that she is suffering from abdominal cramp not a tumor (see the fifth selection, "Abdominal Cramps and Pneumonia"). In this instance he offends the professional hierarchy by contravening the opin-ion of Dr. Minchin, a fully qualified physician, and proving that he commands superior expertise; it is considered "indecent for a general practitioner to contradict a physician's diagnosis in that open manner." It is one of the salient ironies of *Middlemarch* that Lydgate acquires the reputation of being able to effect a "remarkable cure" (for Nancy's alleged tumor) when the disorder was a minor one that could be resolved by rest and good diet. On the auctioneer, Trumbull, who has pneumonia, Lydgate applies the innovative " 'expectant method' " as well as a thermometer to measure the fever. Satisfied with the treatment, Trumbull spreads word that Lydgate " 'knew a thing or two more than the rest of the doc-tors' "—a testimony that of course only intensifies the other doctors' resentment of him.

Another complaint against Lydgate, and another example of the clash between the old and the new concerns his resistance to dispensing medications, then a normal part of a surgeon's (but not of a physician's) duties (see "The Dispensing of Drugs," the fifth selection). Dispensing drugs was considered manual work, appropriate to the lower ranks of surgeon and apothecary, but beneath the dignity of the physician who is supposed to use his head, not his hands. It is interesting to compare Lydgate with Trollope's Dr. Thorne on this matter. Both earn their fellow practitioners' censure for breaking with the conventions, although they do so in opposite directions, as it were. Dr. Thorne, as a graduated physician, is not supposed to dispense drugs, but does so in a rural area for his patients' convenience, whereas Lydgate, a surgeon, refuses to fulfill an obligation expected of him. These parallel incidents are telling evidence of the force of hierarchical institutions in the mid-nineteenth-century British medical system. Lydgate's stand gives rise to the rumor that he does not believe in the effectiveness of medications. Again ahead of his time, he is aware of the dangers of overmedication, particularly with the almost poisonous doses often used in an attempt to attain a cure in what was known as "heroic" medicine. Lydgate is also championing a principle: since surgeons were prohibited from treating internal diseases (but actually did, as Lydgate's work shows), they could not claim payment for such activity, and instead would submit "long bills for draughts, boluses, and mixtures." Lydgate's resistance to excessive medications is sound, honest practice, but it transgresses conventions and expectations, and so offends both his clientele and his fellow medical men in the town.

Still, Lydgate does have a following in Middlemarch among those who appreciate both his expertise and his sensitivity. He shows astute psychological judgment of the amount of information each person can tolerate as well as the ability to impart bad news with tact (see "Facing the Truth," the sixth selection). He decides of his own volition and contrary to the then customary norms that Dorothea should be told of her husband's very precarious state of health, including the possibility of sudden death (which does indeed occur). He follows this course of action because he wants to spare her later regrets. He speaks in a gentle, kindly manner, yet his empathy for her predicament does not prevent him from answering forthrightly the questions she poses. Similarly, when Casaubon himself later summons him, he is equally frank in response to the patient's request "to know the truth without reservation," though again his openness is tempered with caution and circumspection. On the other hand, Lydgate recognizes Mrs. Vincy as too volatile ("convulsive") to stand the truth about her son's dangerous fever. He offers her comfort and support, and recruits her to help in practical ways so as to make her feel useful and to stop her frenzied effusiveness. These diversified examples illustrate Lydgate's flexibility in the ethics of truth-telling.

Despite his diagnostic and therapeutic successes and his psychological acumen, which win him the admiration of the more progressive citizens of Middlemarch, in the long run Lydgate's nonconformity arouses growing opposition. His refusal to dispense drugs, his contravention of other medical men's diagnoses (including physicians'), his advocacy of a fever wing in the new hospital, his treatment of internal diseases all provoke resistance to him both within the profession and among the more ignorant of the populace. Added to these objections is the anxiety expressed by Mrs. Dollop, the landlady of the inn, that Lydgate will kill his patients off in order to obtain corpses to dissect (see the last selection, "Gathering Opposition"). This bizarre fear can be understood only in light of the legal circumstances in Britain at the time. While autopsies were allowed in France, thus making possible the exploration of pathological anatomy, in England they were banned until the Anatomy Act of 1832 (just before the close of the novel's action) sanctioned the lawful acquisition of corpses for dissection. Previously graves had sometimes been robbed and corpses sold for medical research. The notorious case of Burke and Hare is mentioned: they had murdered fifteen people to satisfy the demand for medical specimens.

Middlemarch is a central text for the literature about medicine in the nineteenth century because it gives such a vivid picture of the clash between the old ways of practicing medicine and the new scientific model represented by Lydgate. His superior knowledge and better treatments do not ultimately neutralize the fears, prejudices, ingrained habits, and irrational suspicions of most of the town's inhabitants. His "foreign" methods and his advocacy of reform scare the majority of his patients and are perceived as a threat by the town's old-fashioned practitioners. Nowhere is the conflict between medical progress and social reality articulated with as much sharpness as in the clash between Lydgate and Middlemarch. Lydgate contributes to his own downfall through certain flaws in his character and his poor judgment in marrying a pretty, willful, extravagant young woman who plunges him deep into debt. Eventually he leaves Middlemarch to attend to the wealthy in London and at fashionable watering-places. He dies in middle age, disappointed in himself because he has not fulfilled his potential, let alone his ideals.

Middlemarch raises a number of perplexing questions. Could Lydgate have prevented stark confrontations by more tactful behavior toward his peers/rivals in the town? Ought he have tempered his idealism with a greater consideration for the dominant social realities of the time and place? To what extent do patients command the capacity to assess the worth of a physician's advice, especially as medicine became increasingly imbued with science?. Are the citizens of Middlemarch just too entrenched in their accustomed ways to do justice to Lydgate? In our hyperscientific/technological age, how well equipped are we to set about making valid judgments?

A Conflict of Opinions

George Eliot

Mr Lydgate had the medical accomplishment of looking perfectly grave whatever nonsense was talked to him, and his dark steady eyes gave him impressiveness as a listener. He was as little as possible like the lamented Hicks [a recently deceased practitioner in the area], especially in a certain careless refinement about his toilette and utterance. Yet Lady Chettam gathered much confidence in him. He confirmed her view of her own constitution as being peculiar, by admitting that all constitutions might be called peculiar, and he did not deny that hers might be more peculiar than others. He did not approve of a too lowering system, including reckless cupping (bleeding), nor, on the other hand, of incessant port-wine and bark. He said "I think so" with an air of so much deference accompanying the insight of agreement, that she formed the most cordial opinion of his talents.

"I am quite pleased with your *protege*," she said to Mr Brooke before going away.

"My protege? Dear me!—who is that?" said Mr Brooke.

"This young Lydgate, the new doctor. He seems to me to understand his profession admirably."

"Oh, Lydgate! he is not my *protege*, you know; only I knew an uncle of his who sent me a letter about him. However, I think he is likely to

From George Eliot, *Middlemarch* (Harmondsworth: Penguin, 1965), pp. 118–119.

be first-rate—has studied in Paris, knew Broussais; has ideas, you know— wants to raise the profession."

"Lydgate has lots of ideas, quite new, about ventilation and diet, that sort of thing," resumed Mr Brooke, after he had handed out Lady Chettam, and had returned to be civil to a group of Middlemarchers.

"Hang it, do you think that is quite sound?—upsetting the old treatment, which has made Englishmen what they are?" said Mr Standish.

"Medical knowledge is at a low ebb among us," said Mr Bulstrode, who spoke in a subdued tone, and had rather a sickly air. "I, for my part, hail the advent of Mr Lydgate. I hope to find good reason for confiding the new hospital to his management."

"That is all very fine," replied Mr Standish, who was not fond of Mr Bulstrode, "if you like him to try experiments on your hospital patients, and kill a few people for charity, I have no objection. But I am not going to hand money out of my purse to have experiments tried on me. I like treatment that has been tested a little."

"Well, you know, Standish, every dose you take is an experiment— an experiment, you know," said Mr Brooke, nodding towards the lawyer.

The New Hospital

George Eliot

"I shall be exceedingly obliged if you will look in on me here occasionally, Mr Lydgate," the banker observed, after a brief pause. "If, as I dare
to hope, I have the privilege of finding you a valuable coadjutor in the
interesting matter of hospital management, there will be many questions
which we shall need to discuss in private. As to the new hospital, which
is nearly finished, I shall consider what you have said about the advantages of the special destination for fevers. The decision will rest with me,
for though Lord Medlicote has given the land and timber for the building, he is not disposed to give his personal attention to the object."

"There are few things better worth the pains in a provincial town
like this," said Lydgate. "A fine fever hospital in addition to the old
infirmary might be the nucleus of a medical school here, when once we
get our medical reforms; and what would do more for medical education
than the spread of such schools over the country? A born provincial man
who has a grain of public spirit as well as a few ideas, should do what
he can to resist the rush of everything that is a little better than common
towards London. Any valid professional aims may often find a freer, if
not a richer field, in the provinces."

One of Lydgate's gifts was a voice habitually deep and sonorous, yet
capable of becoming very low and gentle at the right moment. About his

From George Eliot, *Middlemarch* (Harmondsworth: Penguin, 1965), pp. 152–153.

ordinary bearing there was a certain fling, a fearless expectation of success, a confidence in his own powers and integrity much fortified by
contempt for petty obstacles or seductions of which he had had no
experience. But this proud openness was made lovable by an expression
of unaffected good-will. Mr Bulstrode perhaps liked him the better for
the difference between them in pitch and manners; he certainly liked him
the better, as Rosamond did, for being a stranger in Middlemarch. One
can begin so many things with a new person!—even begin to be a better
man.

"I shall rejoice to furnish your zeal with fuller opportunities," Mr
Bulstrode answered; "I mean, by confiding to you the superintendence
of my new hospital, should a maturer knowledge favour that issue, for
I am determined that so great an object shall not be shackled by our two
physicians. Indeed, I am encouraged to consider your advent to this
town as a gracious indication that a more manifest blessing is now to be
awarded to my efforts, which have hitherto been much withstood. With
regard to the old infirmary, we have gained the initial point—I mean
your election. And now I hope you will not shrink from incurring a
certain amount of jealousy and dislike from your professional brethren by
presenting yourself as a reformer."

"I will not profess bravery," said Lydgate, smiling, "but I acknowledge a good deal of pleasure in fighting, and I should not care for my
profession, if I did not believe that better methods were to be found and
enforced there as well as everywhere else."

"The standard of that profession is low in Middlemarch, my dear
sir," said the banker. "I mean in knowledge and skill; not in social status,
for our medical men are most of them connected with respectable townspeople here. My own imperfect health has induced me to give some
attention to those palliative resources which the divine mercy has placed
within our reach. I have consulted eminent men in the metropolis, and
I am painfully aware of the backwardness under which medical treatment
labours in our provincial districts."

"Yes;—with our present medical rules and education, one must be
satisfied now and then to meet with a fair practitioner. As to all the
higher questions which determine the starting-point of a diagnosis—as
to the philosophy of medical evidence—any glimmering of these can only
come from a scientific culture of which country practitioners have usually
no more notion than the man in the moon."

Lydgate's Ideals

George Eliot

Lydgate did not mean to be one of those failures, and there was the better hope of him because his scientific interest soon took the form of a professional enthusiasm: he had a youthful belief in his bread-winning work, not to be stifled by that initiation in makeshift called his 'prentice days; and he carried to his studies in London, Edinburgh, and Paris, the conviction that the medical profession as it might be was the finest in the world; presenting the most perfect interchange between science and art; offering the most direct alliance between intellectual conquest and the social good. Lydgate's nature demanded this combination: he was an emotional creature, with a flesh-and-blood sense of fellowship which withstood all the abstractions of special study. He cared not only for "cases," but for John and Elizabeth, especially Elizabeth.

There was another attraction in his profession: it wanted reform, and gave a man an opportunity for some indignant resolve to reject its venal decorations and other humbug, and to be the possessor of genuine though undemanded qualifications. He went to study in Paris with the determination that when he came home again he would settle in some provincial town as a general practitioner, and resist the irrational severance between medical and surgical knowledge in the interest of his own scientific pursuits, as well as of the general advance: he would keep away from the range of London intrigues, jealousies, and social truckling and

From George Eliot, *Middlemarch* (Harmondsworth: Penguin, 1965), pp. 174–178.

win celebrity, however slowly, as Jenner had done, by the independent value of his work. For it must be remembered that this was a dark period; and in spite of venerable colleges which used great efforts to secure purity of knowledge by making it scarce, and to exclude error by a rigid exclusiveness in relation to fees and appointments, it happened that very ignorant young gentlemen were promoted in town, and many more got a legal right to practise over large areas in the country. Also, the high standard held up to the public mind by the College of Physicians, which gave medical instruction obtained by graduates of Oxford and Cambridge, did not hinder quackery from having an excellent time of it; for since professional practice chiefly consisted in giving a great many drugs, the public inferred that it might be better off with more drugs still, if they could only be got cheaply, and hence swallowed large cubic measures of physic prescribed by unscrupulous ignorance which had taken no degrees. Considering that statistics had not yet embraced a calculation as to the number of ignorant or canting doctors which absolutely must exist in the teeth of all changes, it seemed to Lydgate that a change in the units was the most direct mode of changing the numbers. He meant to be a unit who would make a certain amount of difference towards that spreading change which would one day tell appreciably upon the averages, and in the mean time have the pleasure of making an advantageous difference to the viscera of his own patients. But he did not simply aim at a more genuine kind of practice than was common. He was ambitious of a wider effect: he was fired with the possibility that he might work out the proof of an anatomical conception and make a link in the chain of discovery.

Does it seem incongruous to you that a Middlemarch surgeon should dream of himself as a discoverer? Most of us, indeed, know little of the great originators until they have been lifted up among the constellations and already rule our fates. But that Herschel, for example, who "broke the barriers of the heavens," did he not once play a provincial church-organ, and give music-lessons to stumbling pianists? Each of those Shining Ones had to walk on the earth among neighbours who perhaps thought much more of his gait and his garments than of anything which was to give him a title to everlasting fame: each of them had his little local personal history sprinkled with small temptations and sordid cares, which made the retarding friction of his course towards final companionship with the immortals. Lydgate was not blind to the dangers of such friction, but he had plenty of confidence in his resolution to avoid it as far as possible; being seven-and-twenty, he felt himself experienced. And he was not going to have his vanities provoked by contact with the showy worldly successes of the capital, but to live among people who could hold no rivalry with that pursuit of a great idea which was to be a twin object with assisuous practice of his profession. There was fascination in the hope that the two purposes would illuminate each other: the careful observation and inference which was his daily work, the use of the lens to further his judgment in special cases, would further his thought as an instrument of larger inquiry. Was not this the typical preeminence of his profession? He would be a good Middlemarch doctor, and by that very means keep himself in the track of far-reaching investigation. On one point he may fairly claim approval at this particular stage of his career: he did not mean to imitate those philanthropic models who make a profit out of poisonous pickles to support themselves while they are exposing adulteration, or hold shares in a gambling-hell that they may have leisure to represent the cause of public morality. He intended to begin in his own case some particular reforms which were quite certainly within his reach, and much less of a problem than the demonstrating of an anatomical conception. One of these reforms was to act stoutly on the strength of a recent legal decision, and simply prescribe, without dispensing drugs or taking percentage from druggists. This was an innovation for one who had chosen to adopt the style of general practitioner in a country town, and would be felt as offensive criticism by his professional brethren. But Lydgate meant to innovate in his treatment also, and he was wise enough to see that the best security for his practising honestly according to his belief was to get rid of systematic temptations to the contrary.

Perhaps that was a more cheerful time for observers and theorisers than the present; we are apt to think it the finest era of the world when America was beginning to be discovered, when a bold sailor, even if he were wrecked, might alight on a new kingdom; and about 1829 the dark territories of Pathology were a fine America for a spirited young adventurer. Lydgate was ambitious above all to contribute towards enlarging the scientific, rational basis of his profession. The more he became interested in special questions of disease, such as the nature of fever or fevers, the more keenly he felt the need for that fundamental knowledge of structure which just at the beginning of the century had been illuminated by the brief and glorious career of Bichat, who died when be was only one-and-thirty, but, like another Alexander, left a realm large enough for many heirs. That great Frenchman first carried out the conception that living bodies, fundamentally considered, are not associations of organs which can be understood by studying them first apart, and then as it were federally; but must be regarded as consisting of certain primary webs or tissues, out of which the various organs—brain, heart, lungs, and so on—are compacted, as the various accommodations of a house are built up in various proportions of wood, iron, stone, brick, zinc, and the rest, each material having its peculiar composition and proportions. No man, one sees, can understand and estimate the entire structure or its parts—what are its frailties and what its repairs, without knowing the nature of the materials. And the conception wrought out by Bichat, with his detailed study of the different tissues, acted necessarily on medical questions as the turning of gaslight would act on a dim, oil-lit street, showing new connections and hitherto hidden facts of structure which must be taken into account in considering the symptoms of maladies and the action of medicaments. But results which depend on human con-science and intelligence work slowly, and now at the end of 1829, most medical practice was still strutting or shambling along the old paths, and there was still scientific work to be done which might have seemed to be a direct sequence of Bichat's. This great seer did not go beyond the consideration of the tissues as ultimate facts in the living organism, marking the limit of anatomical analysis; but it was open to another mind to say, have not these structures some common basis from which they have all started, as your sarsnet, gauze, net, satin velvet from the raw cocoon? Here would be another light, as of oxy-hydrogen, showing the very grain of things, and revising all former explanations. Of this sequence to Bichat's work, already vibrating along many currents of the European mind, Lydgate was enamoured; he longed to demonstrate the more intimate relations of living structure, and help to define men's thought more accurately after the true order. The work had not yet been done, but only prepared for those who knew how to use the preparation. What was the primitive tissue? In that way Lydgate put the question—not quite in the way required by the awaiting answer; but such missing of the right word befalls many seekers. And he counted on quiet intervals to be watchfully seized, for taking up the threads of investigation—on many hints to be won from diligent application, not only of the scalpel, but of the microscope which research had begun to use again with new enthu-siasm of reliance. Such was Lydgate's plan for his future: to do good small work for Middlemarch, and great work for the world.

A Case of Typhoid Fever

George Eliot

But Fred did not go to Stone Court the next day, for reasons that were quite peremptory. From those visits to unsanitary Houndsley streets in search of Diamond, he had brought back not only a bad bargain in horse-flesh, but the further misfortunee of some ailment which for a day or two had seemed mere depression and headache, but which got so much worse when he returned from his visit to Stone Court that, going into the dining-room, he threw himself on the sofa, and in answer to his mother's anxious question, said, "I feel very ill: I think you must send for Wrench."

Wrench came but did not apprehend anything serious, spoke of a "slight derangement," and did not speak of coming again on the morrow. He had a due value for the Vincys' house, but the wariest men are apt to be a little dulled by routine, and on worried mornings will sometimes go through their business with the zest of the daily bell-ringer. Mr Wrench was a small, neat, bilious man,—with a well-dressed wig: he had a laborious practice, an irascible temper, a lymphatic wife and seven children; and he was already rather late before setting out on a four-miles' drive to meet Dr Minchin on the other side of Tipton, the decease of Hicks, a rural practitioner, having increased Middlemarch practice in that direction. Great statesmen err, and why not small medical men? Mr Wrench did not neglect sending the usual white parcels, which this time

From George Eliot, *Middlemarch* (Harmondsworth: Penguin, 1965), pp. 292–294.

had black and drastic contents. Their effect was not alleviating to poor
Fred, who, however, unwilling as he said to believe that he was "in for
an illness," rose at his usual easy hour the next morning and went
downstairs meaning to breakfast, but succeeded in nothing but in sitting
and shivering by the fire. Mr Wrench was again sent for, but was gone
on his rounds, and Mrs Vincy seeing her darling's changed looks and
general misery, began to cry and said she would send for Dr Sprague.

"Oh, nonsense, mother! It's nothing," said Fred, putting out his hot
dry hand to her, "I shall soon be all right. I must have taken cold in that
nasty damp ride."

"Mamma!" said Rosamond, who was seated near the window (the
dining-room windows looked on that highly respectable street called
Lowick Gate), "there is Mr Lydgate, stopping to speak to some one. If
I were you I would call him in. He has cured Ellen Bulstrode. They say
he cures every one."

Mrs Vincy sprang to the window and opened it in an instant, thinking only of Fred and not of medical etiquette. Lydgate was only two
yards off on the other side of some iron palisading, and turned round at
the sudden sound of the sash, before she called to him. In two minutes
he was in the room, and Rosamond went out, after waiting just long
enough to show a pretty anxiety conflicting with her sense of what was
becoming.

Lydgate had to hear a narrative in which Mrs Vincy's mind insisted
with remarkable instinct on every point of minor importance, especially
on what Mr Wrench had said and had not said about coming again. That
there might be an awkward affair with Wrench, Lydgate saw at once; but
the case was serious enough to make him dismiss that consideration: he
was convinced that Fred was in the pink-skinned stage of typhoid fever,
and that he had taken just the wrong medicines. He must go to bed
immediately, must have a regular nurse, and various appliances and pre-
cautions must be used, about which Lydgate was particular. Poor Mrs
Vincy's terror at these indications of danger found vent in such words as
came most easily. She thought it "very ill usage on the part of Mr
Wrench, who had attended their house so many years in preference to
Mr Peacock, though Mr Peacock was equally a friend. Why Mr Wrench
should neglect her children more than others, she could not for the life
of her understand. He had not neglected Mrs. Larcher's when they had
the measles, nor indeed would Mrs Vincy have wished that he should.
And if anything should happen . . ."

Here poor Mrs Vincy's spirit quite broke down, and her Niobe-
throat and good-humoured face were sadly convulsed. This was in the

hall out of Fred's hearing, but Rosamond had opened the drawing-room door, and now came forward anxiously. Lydgate apologised for Mr Wrench, said that the symptoms yesterday might have been disguising, and that this form of fever was very equivocal in its beginnings: he would go immediately to the druggist's and have a prescription made up in order to lose no time, but he would write to Mr Wrench and tell him what had been done.

But you must come again—you must go on attending Fred. I can't have my boy left to anybody who may come or not. I bear nobody ill-will, thank God, and Mr Wrench saved me in the pleurisy, but he'd better have let me die—if—if—"

"I will meet Mr Wrench here, then, shall I?" said Lydgate, really believing that Wrench was not well prepared to deal wisely with a case of this kind.

"Pray make that arrangement, Mr Lydgate," said Rosamond, coming to her mother's aid, and supporting her arm to lead her away.

Dispensing of Drugs

George Eliot

But irrational reproaches were easier to bear than the sense of being instructed, or rather the sense that a younger man, like Lydgate, inwardly considered him in need of instruction, for "in point of fact," Mr Wrench afterwards said, Lydgate paraded flighty, foreign notions, which would not wear. He swallowed his ire for the moment, but he afterwards wrote to decline further attendance in the case. The house might be a good one, but Mr Wrench was not going to truckle to anybody on a professional matter. He reflected, with much probability on his side, that Lydgate would by-and-by be caught tripping too, and that his ungentlemanly attempts to discredit the sale of drugs by his professional brethren would by-and-by recoil on himself. He threw out biting remarks on Lydgate's tricks, worthy only of a quack, to get himself a factitious reputation with credulous people. That cant about cures was never got up by sound practitioners.

From George Eliot, *Middlemarch* (Harmondsworth: Penguin, 1965), pp. 295–296.

Abdominal Cramps and Pneumonia

George Eliot

Mrs Larcher having just become charitably concerned about alarming symptoms in her charwoman, when Dr Minchin called, asked him to see her then and there, and to give her a certificate for the Infirmary; where-upon after examination he wrote a statement of the case as one of tumour, and recommended the bearer Nancy Nash as an outpatient. Nancy, calling at the home on her way to the Infirmary, allowed the staymaker and his wife, in whose attic she lodged, to read Dr Minchin's paper, and by this means became a subject of compassionate conversation in the neighbouring shops of Churchyard Lane as being afflicted with a tumour at first declared to be as large and hard as a duck's egg, but later in the day to be about the size of "your fist." Most hearers agreed that it would have to be cut out, but one had known of oil and another of "squitchineal" as adequate to soften and reduce any lump in the body when taken enough of into the inside—the oil by gradually "soopling," the squitchineal by eating away.

Meanwhile when Nancy presented herself at the Infirmary, it hap-pened to be one of Lydgate's days there. After questioning and exam-ining her, Lydgate said to the house-surgeon in an undertone, "It's not tumour: it's cramp." He ordered her a blister and some steel mixture,

From George Eliot, *Middlemarch* (Harmondsworth: Penguin, 1965), pp. 489–491.

125

and told her to go home and rest, giving her at the same time a note to Mrs Larcher, who, she said, was her best employer, to testify that she was in need of good food.

But by-and-by Nancy, in her attic, became portentously worse, the supposed tumour having indeed given way to the blister, but only wandered to another region with angrier pain. The staymaker's wife went to fetch Lydgate, and he continued for a fortnight to attend Nancy in her own home, until under his treatment she got quite well and went to work again. But the case continued to be described as one of tumour in Churchyard Lane and other streets—nay, by Mrs Larcher also; for when Lydgate's remarkable cure was mentioned to Dr Minchin, he naturally did not like to say, "The case was not one of tumour, and I was mistaken in describing it as such," but answered, "Indeed! ah! I saw it was a surgical case, not of a fatal kind." He had been inwardly annoyed, however, when he had asked at the Infirmary about the woman he had recommended two days before, to hear from the house-surgeon, a youngster who was not sorry to vex Minchin with impunity, exactly what had occurred: he privately pronounced that it was indecent in a general practitioner to contradict a physician's diagnosis in that open manner, and afterwards agreed with Wrench that Lydgate was disagreeably inattentive to etiquette. Lydgate did not make the affair a ground for valuing himself or (very particularly) despising Minchin, such rectification of misjudgments often happening among men of equal qualifications. But report took up the amazing case of the tumour, not clearly distinguished from cancer, and considered the more awful for being of the wandering sort; till much prejudice against Lydgate's method as to drugs was overcome by the proof of his marvellous skill in the speedy restoration of Nancy Nash after she had been rolling and rolling in agonies from the presence of a tumour both hard and obstinate, but nevertheless compelled to yield.

How could Lydgate help himself? It is offensive to tell a lady when she is expressing her amazement at your skill, that she is altogether mistaken and rather foolish in her amazement. And to have entered into the nature of diseases would only have added to his breaches of medical propriety. Thus he had to wince under a promise of success given by that ignorant praise which misses every valid quality.

In the case of a more conspicuous patient, Mr Borthrop Trumbull, Lydgate was conscious of having shown himself something better than an everyday doctor, though here too it was an equivocal advantage that he won. The eloquent auctioneer was seized with pneumonia, and having been a patient of Mr Peacock's, sent for Lydgate, whom he had expressed his intention to patronise. Mr Trumbull was a robust man, a good subject for trying the expectant theory upon—watching the course of an interesting disease when left as much as possible to itself, so that the stages might be noted for future guidance; and from the air with which he described his sensations Lydgate surmised that he would like to be taken into his medical man's confidence, and be represented as a partner in his own cure. The auctioneer heard, without much surprise, that his was a constitution which (always with due watching) might be left to itself, so as to offer a beautiful example of a disease with all its phases seen in clear delineation, and that he probably had the rare strength of mind voluntarily to become the test of a rational procedure, and thus make the disorder of his pulmonary functions a general benefit to society.

Mr Trumbull acquiesced at once, and entered strongly into the view that an illness of his was no ordinary occasion for medical science. "Never fear, sir; you are not speaking to one who is altogether ignorant of the *vis medicatrix* (medical power)," said he, with his usual superiority of expression, made rather pathetic by difficulty of breathing. And he went without shrinking through his abstinence from drugs, much sustained by application of the thermometer which implied the importance of his temperature, by the sense that he furnished objects for the microscope, and by learning many new words which seemed suited to the dignity of his secretions. For Lydgate was acute enough to indulge him with a little technical talk.

It may be imagined that Mr Trumbull rose from his couch with a disposition to speak of an illness in which he had manifested the strength of his mind as well as constitution; and he was not backward in awarding credit to the medical man who had discerned the quality of patient he had to deal with. The auctioneer was not an ungenerous man, and liked to give others their due, feeling that he could afford it. He had caught the words "expectant method," and rang chimes on this and other learned phrases to accompany the assurance that Lydgate "knew a thing or two more than the rest of the doctors—was far better versed in the secrets of his profession than the majority of his compeers."

Facing the Truth

George Eliot

Lydgate had determined on speaking to Dorothea. She had not been present while her uncle was throwing out his pleasant suggestions as to the mode in which life at Lowick might be enlivened, but she was usually by her husband's side, and the unaffected signs of intense anxiety in her face and voice about whatever touched his mind or health, made a drama which Lydgate was inclined to watch. He said to himself that he was only doing right in telling her the truth about her husband's probable future, but he certainly thought also that it would be interesting to talk confidentially with her. A medical man likes to make psychological observations, and sometimes in the pursuit of such studies is too easily tempted into momentous prophecy which life and death easily set at nought. Lydgate had often been satirical on this gratuitous prediction, and he meant now to be guarded.

He asked for Mrs Casaubon, but being told that she was out walking, he was going away, when Dorothea and Celia appeared, both glowing from their struggle with the March wind. When Lydgate begged to speak with her alone, Dorothea opened the library door which happened to be the nearest, thinking of nothing at the moment but what he might have to say about Mr Casaubon. It was the first time she had entered this room since her husband had been taken ill, and the servant had chosen

From George Eliot, *Middlemarch* (Harmondsworth: Penguin, 1965), pp. 321–323, 459–461.

128

not to open the shutters. But there was light enough to read by from the narrow upper panes of the windows.

"You will not mind this sombre light," said Dorothea, standing in the middle of the room. "Since you forbade books, the library has been out of the question. But Mr Casaubon will soon be here again, I hope. Is he not making progress?"

"Yes, much more rapid progress than I at first expected. Indeed, he is already nearly in his usual state of health."

"You do not fear that the illness will return?" said Dorothea, whose quick ear had detected some significance in Lydgate's tone.

"Such cases are peculiarly difficult to pronounce upon," said Lydgate. "The only point on which I can be confident is that it will be desirable to be very watchful on Mr Casaubon's account lest he should in any way strain his nervous power."

"I beseech you to speak quite plainly," said Dorothea, in an imploring tone. "I cannot bear to think that there might be something which I did not know, and which, if I had known it, would have made me act differently." The words came out like a cry: it was evident that they were the voice of some mental experience which lay not very off.

"Sit down," she added, placing herself on the nearest chair, and throwing off her bonnet and gloves, with an instinctive discarding of formality where a great question of destiny was concerned.

"What you say now justifies my own view," said Lydgate. "I think it is one's function as a medical man to hinder regrets of that sort as far as possible. But I beg you to observe that Mr Casaubon's case is precisely of the kind in which the issue is most difficult to pronounce upon. He may possibly live for fifteen years or more, without much worse health than he has had hitherto."

Dorothea had turned very pale, and when Lydgate paused she said in a low voice, "You mean if we are very careful."

"Yes—careful against mental agitation of all kinds, and against excessive application."

"He would be miserable, if he had to give up his work," said Dorothea, with a quick prevision of that wretchedness.

"I am aware of that. The only course is to try by all means, direct and indirect, to moderate and vary his occupations. With a happy concurrence of circumstances, there is, as I said, no immediate danger from that affection of the heart which I believe to have been the cause of his late attack. On the other hand, it is possible that the disease may develop itself more rapidly: it is one of those cases in which death is sometimes sudden. Nothing should be neglected which might be affected by such an issue."

There was silence for a few moments, while Dorothea sat as if she had been turned to marble, though the life within her was so intense that her mind had never before swept in brief time over an equal range of scenes and motives.

"Help me, pray," she said, at last, in the same low voice as before. "Tell me what I can do."

"What do you think of foreign travel? You have been lately in Rome, I think."

The memories which made this resource utterly hopeless were a new current that shook Dorothea out of her pallid immobility.

"Oh, that would not do—that would be worse than anything," she said with a more childlike despondency, while the tears rolled down. "Nothing will be of any use that he does not enjoy."

"I wish that I could have spared you this pain," said Lydgate, deeply touched, yet wondering about her marriage. Women just like Dorothea had not entered into his traditions.

"It was right of you to tell me. I thank you for telling me the truth."

"I wish you to understand that I shall not say anything to enlighten Mr Casaubon himself. I think it desirable for him to know nothing more than that he must not overwork himself, and must observe certain rules. Anxiety of any kind would be precisely the most unfavourable condition for him."

Lydgate rose, and Dorothea mechanically rose at the same time, unclasping her cloak and throwing it off as if it stifled her.

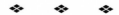

When Lydgate entered the Yew-Tree Walk he saw Mr Casaubon slowly receding with his hands behind him according to his habit, and his head bent forward. It was a lovely afternoon; the leaves from the lofty limes were falling silently across the sombre evergreens, while the lights and shadows slept side by side: there was no sound but the cawing of the rooks, which to the accustomed ear is a lullaby, or that last solemn lullaby, a dirge. Lydgate, conscious of an energetic frame in its prime, felt some compassion when the figure which he was likely soon to overtake turned round, and in advancing towards him showed more markedly than ever the signs of premature age—the student's bent shoulders, the emaciated limbs, and the melancholy lines of the mouth. "Poor fellow," he thought, "some men with his years are like lions; one can tell nothing of their age except that they are full grown."

"Mr Lydgate," said Mr Casaubon, with his invariably polite air, "I am exceedingly obliged to you for your punctuality. We will, if you please, carry on our conversation in walking to and fro."

"I hope your wish to see me is not due to the return of unpleasant symptoms," said Lydgate, filling up a pause.

"Not immediately—no. In order to account for that wish I must mention—what it were otherwise needless to refer to—that my life, on all collateral accounts insignificant, derives a possible importance from the incompleteness of labours which have extended through all its best years. In short, I have long had on hand a work which I would fain leave behind me in such a state, at least, that it might be committed to the press by others. Were I assured that this is the utmost I can reasonably expect, that assurance would be a useful circumscription of my attempts, and a guide in both the positive and negative determination of my course."

Here Mr Casaubon paused, removed one hand from his back and thrust it between the buttons of his single-breasted coat. To a mind largely instructed in the human destiny hardly anything could be more interesting than the inward conflict implied in his formal measured address, delivered with the usual sing-song and motion of the head. Nay, are there many situations more sublimely tragic than the struggle of the soul with the demand to renounce a work which has been all the significance of its life—a significance which is to vanish as the waters which come and go where no man has need of them? But there was nothing to strike others as sublime about Mr Casaubon, and Lydgate, who had some contempt at hand for futile scholarship, felt a little amusement mingling with his pity. He was at present too ill acquainted with disaster to enter into the pathos of a lot where everything is below the level of tragedy except the passionate egoism of the sufferer.

"You refer to the possible hindrances from want of health?" he said, wishing to help forward Mr Casaubon's purpose, which seemed to be clogged by some hesitation.

"I do. You have not implied to me that the symptoms which—I am bound to testify—you watched with scrupulous care, were those of a fatal disease. But were it so, Mr Lydgate, I should desire to know the truth without reservation, and I appeal to you for an exact statement of your conclusions: I request it as a friendly service. If you can tell me that my life is not threatened by anything else than ordinary casualties, I shall rejoice, on grounds which I have already indicated. If not, knowledge of the truth is even more important to me."

"Then I can no longer hesitate as to my course," said Lydgate; "but the first thing I must impress on you is that my conclusions are doubly uncertain-uncertain not only because of my fallibility, but because diseases of the heart are eminently difficult to found predictions on. In any case, one can hardly increase appreciably the tremendous uncertainty of life."

Mr Casaubon winced perceptibly, but bowed.

"I believe that you are suffering from what is called fatty degeneration of the heart, a disease which was first divined and explored by Laennec, the man who gave us the stethoscope, not so very many years ago. A good deal of experience—a more lengthened observation—is wanted on the subject. But after what you have said, it is my duty to tell you that death from this disease is often sudden. At the same time, no such result can be predicted. Your condition may be consistent with a tolerably comfortable life for another fifteen years, or even more. I could add no information to this, beyond anatomical or medical details, which would leave expectation at precisely the same point."

Lydgate's instinct was fine enough to tell him that plain speech, quite free from ostentatious caution, would be felt by Mr Casaubon as a tribute of respect.

"I thank you, Mr Lydgate," said Mr Casaubon, after a moment's pause. "One thing more I have still to ask: did you communicate what you have now told me to Mrs Casaubon?"

"Partly—I mean, as to the possible issues." Lydgate was going to explain why he had told Dorothea, but Mr Casaubon, with an unmistakable desire to end the conversation, waved his hand slightly, and said again, "I thank you," proceeding to remark on the rare beauty of the day.

Gathering Opposition

George Eliot

That opposition to the New Fever Hospital which Lydgate had sketched to Dorothea was, like other oppositions, to be viewed in many different lights. He regarded it as a mixture of jealousy and dunderheaded prejudice. Mr Bulstrode saw in it not only medical jealousy but a determination to thwart himself, prompted mainly by a hatred of that vital religion of which he had striven to be an effectual lay representative—a hatred which certainly found pretexts apart from religion such as were only too easy to find in the entanglements of human action. These might be called the ministerial views. But oppositions have the illimitable range of objections at command, which need never stop short at the boundary of knowledge, but can draw for ever on the vasts of ignorance. What the opposition in Middlemarch said about the New Hospital and its administration had certainly a great deal of echo in it, for heaven has taken care that everybody shall not be an originator;—but there were differences which represented every social shade between the polished moderation of Dr Minchin and the trenchant assertion of Mrs Dollop, the landlady of the Tankard in Slaughter Lane.

Mrs Dollop became more and more convinced by her own asseveration, that Doctor Lydgate meant to let the people die in the Hospital, if not to poison them, for the sake of cutting them up without saying by your leave or with your leave; for it was a known "fac" that he had

From George Eliot, *Middlemarch* (Harmondsworth: Penguin, 1965), pp. 481–483.

wanted to cut up Mrs Goby, as respectable a woman as any in Parley Street, who had money in trust before her marriage—a poor tale for a doctor, who if he was good for anything should know what was the matter with you before you died, and not want to pry into your inside after you were gone. If that was not reason, Mrs Dollop wished to know what was; but there was a prevalent feeling in her audience that her opinion was a bulwark, and that if it were overthrown there would be no limits to the cutting-up of bodies, as had been well seen in Burke and Hare with their pitch-plaisters—such a hanging business as that was not wanted in Middlemarch!

And let it not be supposed that opinion at the Tankard in Slaughter Lane was unimportant to the medical profession: that old authentic public-house—the original Tankard, known by the name of Dollop's—was the resort of a great Benefit [Insurance] Club, which had some months before put to the vote whether its longstanding medical man, "Doctor Gambit," should not be cashiered in favour of "this Doctor Lydgate," who was capable of performing the most astonishing cures, and rescuing people altogether given up by other practitioners. But the balance had been turned against Lydgate by two members, who for some private reasons held that this power of resuscitating persons as good as dead was an equivocal recommendation, and might interfere with providential favours. In the course of the year, however, there had been a change in the public sentiment, of which the unanimity at Dollop's was an index.

A good deal more than a year ago, before anything was known of Lydgate's skill, the judgments on it had naturally been divided, depending on a sense of likelihood, situated perhaps in the pit of the stomach or in the pineal gland, and differing in its verdicts, but not the less valuable as a guide in the total deficit of evidence. Patients who had chronic diseases or whose lives had long been worn threadbare, like old Featherstone's, had been at once inclined to try him; also, many who did not like paying their doctor's bills, thought agreeably of opening an account with a new doctor and sending for him without stint if the children's temper wanted a dose, occasions when the old practitioners were often crusty; and all persons thus inclined to employ Lydgate held it likely that he was clever. Some considered that he might do more than others "where there was liver; at least there would be no harm in getting a few bottles of "stuff" from him, since if these proved useless it would still be possible to return to the Purifying Pills, which kept you alive, if they did not remove the yellowness. But these were people of minor importance. Good Middlemarch families were of course not going to change their doctor without reason shown; and everybody who had employed Mr Peacock did not feel obliged to accept a new man merely in the character of his successor, objecting that he was "not likely to be equal to Peacock."

But Lydgate had not been long in the town before there were particulars enough reported of him to breed much more specific expectations and to intensify differences into partisanship; some of the particulars being of that impressive order of which the significance is entirely hidden, like a statistical amount without a standard of comparison, but with a note of exclamation at the end. The cubic feet of oxygen yearly swallowed bv a full-grown man—what a shudder they might have created in some Middlemarch circles! "Oxygen! nobody knows what that may be—is it any wonder the cholera has got to Dantzic? And yet there are people who say quarantine is no good!"

One of the facts quickly rumoured was that Lydgate did not dispense drugs. This was offensive both to the physicians whose exclusive distinction seemed infringed on, and to the surgeon-apothecaries with whom he ranged himself; and only a little while before, they might have counted on having the law on their side against a man who without calling himself a London-made M.D. dared to ask for pay except as a charge on drugs. But Lydgate had not been experienced enough to foresee that his new course would be even more offensive to the laity; and to Mr Mawmsey, an important grocer in the Top Market, who, though not one of his patients, questioned him in an affable manner on the subject, he was injudicious enough to give a hasty popular explanation of his reasons, pointing out to Mr Mawmsey that it must lower the character of practitioners, and be a constant injury to the public, if their only mode of getting paid for their work was by their making out long bills for draughts, boluses, and mixtures.

6

The Laboratory and Its Products

An Introduction to Selections from Robert Louis Stevenson's Dr. Jekyll and Mr. Hyde

Robert Louis Stevenson (1850–1894), a Scottish novelist, poet, and essayist, wrote a number of well-known works including *Treasure Island* (1883), *Kidnapped* (1886), and *Dr. Jekyll and Mr. Hyde* (1886). His essay collection, *Travels with a Donkey in the Cevennes* (1879), is the product of an attempt to treat the tuberculosis from which he suffered by fresh air in the mountains. After marrying an American in 1880, he settled in 1888 in the milder climate of Samoa, where he died of tuberculosis. His lengthy illness gave him personal experience of the world of medicine.

The full title of the story which was his greatest success and is usually known as just *Dr. Jekyll and Mr. Hyde* is *The Strange Case of Dr. Jekyll and Mr. Hyde*. "Case" carries a double meaning here, referring to both a medical and a legal case. Stevenson had completed training as a lawyer, although he never actually practiced his profession. But the narrator of *Dr. Jekyll and Mr. Hyde* is the lawyer, Mr. Utterson, who has been charged by a friend to investigate the criminal activities of a Mr. Hyde, who is terrorizing an area of London, and who eventually commits a murder. What makes the case so mystifying from the outset is that Mr. Hyde pays off a victim with a genuine check he signs on a reputable bank in the name of a highly respected figure (see the first selection, "The Deliquent Mr. Hyde and His Check"). That person turns out to be the eminent physician, Henry Jekyll, M.D., D.C.L., LL.D., F.R.S. (Doctor of Medicine, Doctor of Civil Law, Doctor of Law, Fellow of the Royal

Society), who on his death leaves all his possessions to his friend, Edward Hyde.

Dr. Jekyll and Mr. Hyde can be read from a number of different angles. Most obviously it is a detective story: Mr. Utterson is determined to unravel the puzzling connection that appears to exist between the criminal Mr. Hyde and the honored Dr. Jekyll. A series of perplexing "incidents," as three of the sections are entitled, heighten the tension. So also does the interpolated "narrative" of Dr. Lanyon, a colleague of Dr. Jekyll, to whom he appeals for help. Letters sent out by Dr. Jekyll play an equally important part; it is in the last of these, in the closing section, "Henry Jekyll's Full Statement," that the mystery is finally solved through Jekyll's own confession. Although readers can make a good guess at the outcome, its actual details still provide a surprising ending to the story.

The identification of Mr. Hyde as coinciding with Dr. Jekyll has supported the most prevalent reading of this tale as one concerned with dual personality. Stevenson shows remarkable, instinctive insight into the workings of split personality at a time when there was little medical understanding of the phenomenon. In this respect the impetus for the story stems more from the mythology of the evil other than from scientific knowledge. Repeated emphasis is placed on the contrast between the "damnable," "wicked," "evil," "inherently malign and villanous" Mr. Hyde and the "proper," indeed "celebrated" Dr. Jekyll. The story's shock effect comes partly from the reader's discovery that they are one and the same person. This immediately raises the question which becomes the central puzzle impelling the narrative: how can this possibly have happened?

Dr. Jekyll and Mr. Hyde has medico-historical implications too that have so far been overshadowed by its horror story aspects; it represents an oblique commentary on the public apprehension of the research laboratory in the later nineteenth century. On his first visit to Dr. Jekyll's home (described in the second selection, "Visits to Dr. Jekyll"), Mr. Utterson at once senses the eeriness of the doctor's "laboratory": he gazes at it not only with "curiosity" but also "with a distasteful sense of strangeness" as he passes through it on his way to the residential quarters upstairs. Earlier the space had been the dissecting-room of a celebrated surgeon, the previous owner of the house; its conversion into a laboratory full of "chemical apparatus" reflects the shift of focus from the pathology foremost in the opening decades of the century to the emphasis on chemistry from mid-century onward. Private, home laboratories such as Dr. Jekyll's, Lydgate's in *Middlemarch*, or the research physician's in Emile Zola's *Le Docteur Pascal* (1893; Doctor Pascal) were becoming rare in the late nineteenth century as research was organized into a group activity. Some institutes were state funded (e.g., the Pasteur in Paris, founded in 1888, and the Koch in Berlin in 1891). The early 1890s were the heyday for the inauguration of research institutes: the Institute for Experimental Medicine in St. Petersburg in 1892, the British Institute of Preventive Medicine in London in 1893, and the Serotherapeutic Institute in Vienna in 1894. It was also in 1892 that the first American laboratories of hygiene opened at the University of Pennsylvania and in New York City as part of its health department, while in 1894 Johns Hopkins University dedicated its William Pepper laboratory. In addition, commercially motivated research laboratories began to appear too, though not until the early twentieth century when the money-making potential of science was becoming evident. A major instance of such a self-financing laboratory is that of Sir Almoth Wright in London; it grew out of a poky basement room in 1902, intent on finding a weed-killer for bacterial farming, to the rather grand enterprise occupying two storys in a spacious modern building where Alexander Fleming stumbled on penicillin in 1928.

Dr. Jekyll's office ("cabinet") is as yet quite simple, fitted with glass cases ("presses") that presumably also hold professional equipment. Despite the domesticity of the fire in the grate and the lamp, the room is pervaded by an aura of unease symbolized by the fog creeping in through the windows. Dr. Jekyll himself looks "deadly sick." The description clearly implies that something is fundamentally amiss. This is confirmed, and the mystery intensified, in the bewildering contrast Mr. Utterson experiences on a subsequent visit to Jekyll's home between the coziness of the tea things and the startling blasphemies, in Jekyll's own handwriting, scribbled into books for which the doctor had always expressed great esteem. Increasingly the chemicals stand out as the fulcrum of the story. Jekyll's extreme eagerness to locate a certain drug conveys his dire distress, and suggests the desperate situation in which he is stranded without it (see the third selection, "Crying Out for the Drug"). That Dr. Jekyll had been engaging for many years in a sequence of experiments emerges from Dr. Lanyon's narrative as he finds the records Dr. Jekyll had been keeping of his scientific work. Like Mr. Utterson, Dr. Lanyon is completely at a loss to understand what has been going on (see "Dr. Jekyll's Experiments," the fourth selection).

The whole horrendous truth comes to light in the statement left by Dr. Jekyll, read by Mr. Utterson after the doctor's death (in the fifth selection, "Dr. Jekyll's Confession"). Although well aware of the danger inherent in his experimentation, Dr. Jekyll admits that "the temptation of a discovery so singular and so profound at last overcame the suggestion of alarm." The drug he had been taking possessed the power to turn his good public self into the hidden evil Mr. Hyde, and back again. Dr. Jekyll could return "to his good qualities seemingly unimpaired" after releasing the depraved Hyde to pursue his life of crime. Until the day came when the drug's restorative transformation fails, and Jekyll remains captive in Hyde's monstrous persona. So ultimately Dr. Jekyll falls victim to his own scientific curiosity, which has driven him on to experiment despite the risks he knows to be involved. He suppresses ethical scruples about his dangerous pursuits because, like Dr. Griffon in Sue's *Les Mystères de Paris*, he becomes intoxicated with the potential of science. Since he conducts his experimentation on himself, not on patients, he is less nefarious than Dr. Griffon except in the crimes committed by Mr. Hyde.

The Strange Case of Dr. Jekyll and Mr. Hyde can therefore be seen as a cautionary tale about the hazards of laboratory experimentation, not merely to those engaged in it but also to those around them. Mr. Hyde's origins in the laboratory are brought out by his being invariably seen to come and go through its door. The figure of Mr. Hyde stands in the literary tradition of the man-made monster, best exemplified by Mary Shelley's *Frankenstein* (1818), but turned in Stevenson's narrative into the embodiment of sheer gratuitous destructiveness. While Jekyll defends the drug as "neither diabolical nor divine" in and of itself, the story shows the evil that can be wrought by a good person through dabbling with chemicals. So the suspicion and fear aroused by laboratory experimentation in the later nineteenth century is given vivid form in Stevenson's sinister tale. The laboratory's potential for evil assumes graphic shape in Mr. Hyde, whereas no mention is made of the good that might accrue from its discoveries. But *Dr. Jekyll and Mr. Hyde* has to be seen in light of its historical moment, at a point when the laboratory was barely beginning to produce therapeutic remedies (e.g., the rabies vaccine in 1885).

Like *Middlemarch*, Stevenson's story uncovers deeply ingrained suspicion of scientific innovation. It shows the difficulty that even a qualified physician may experience in foreseeing the outcome of his experiments. Dr. Jekyll is like the sorcerer's apprentice who cannot control the process he has initiated. This mythological undercurrent endows the story with additional force. The laboratory's pernicious aura is also intensified by association with the black magic of alchemy. It is portrayed not just as a weird, uncanny place of menacing mystery but as a source of iniquity that undermines the orderly fabric of society. This negative literary image is in stark contrast to the idealization of the laboratory as the "true sanctuary" of medicine by the French physician Claude Bernard (1813–1878) in his highly influential *Introduction à l'étude de la médecine expérimentale* (1865; Introduction to the Experimental Study of Medicine [1927]). The social reality of distrust of the laboratory and its products is a graphic illustration of the discrepancy between hopes for medical research and the fears ingrained in public opinion.

Yet *Dr. Jekyll and Mr. Hyde* differs from *Middlemarch* insofar as we are given to understand that the results of Lydgate's work will be to the good of humankind. How were people to distinguish such potentially beneficial scientific work from the disastrous consequences of Dr. Jekyll's research? Is he responsible for Mr. Hyde's crimes? How does Dr. Jekyll's misuse of science differ from that of Bovary and Homais in *Madame Bovary*? Do these literary works help us to understand the fears current in the later nineteenth century that science could be injurious? To what extent do we still harbor reservations about the impact of science and technology?

The Delinquent Mr. Hyde
and His Check

Robert Louis Stevenson

"All at once, I saw two figures: one a little man who was stumping along eastward at a good walk, and the other a girl of maybe eight or ten who was running as hard as she was able down a cross-street. Well, sir, the two ran into one another naturally enough at the corner; and then came the horrible part of the thing; for the man trampled calmly over the child's body and left her screaming on the ground. It sounds nothing to hear, but it was hellish to see. It wasn't like a man; it was like some damned Juggernaut. I gave a view halloa, took to my heels, collared my gentleman, and brought him back to where there was already quite a group about the screaming child. He was perfectly cool and made no resistance, but gave me one look, so ugly that it brought out the sweat on me like running. The people who had turned out were the girl's own family; and pretty soon the doctor, for whom she had been sent, put in his appearance. Well, the child was not much the worse, more frightened, according to the Sawbones; and there you might have supposed would be an end to it. But there was one curious circumstance. I had taken a loathing to my gentleman at first sight. So had the child's family, which was only natural. But the doctor's case was what struck me. He was the usual cut-and-dry

From Robert Louis Stevenson, *Dr. Jekyll and Mr. Hyde* (London: Dent [Everyman], 1962), pp. 5–6.

apothecary, of no particular age and colour, with a strong Edinburgh accent, and about as emotional as a bagpipe. Well, sir, he was like the rest of us: every time he looked at my prisoner, I saw that Sawbones turned sick and white with the desire to kill him. I knew what was in his mind, just as he knew what was in mine; and killing being out of question, we did the next best. We told the man we could and would make such a scandal out of this, should make his name stink from one end of London to the other. If he had any friends or any credit, we undertook that he should lose them. And all the time, as we were pitching it in red hot, we were keeping the women off him as best we could, for they were as wild as harpies. I never saw a circle of such hateful faces, and there was the man in the middle, with a kind of black sneering coolness—frightened too, I could see that—but carrying it off, sir, really like Satan. 'If you choose to make capital out of this accident,' said he, 'I am naturally helpless. No gentleman but wishes to avoid a scene,' says he. 'Name your figure.' Well, we screwed him up to a hundred pounds for the child's family; he would have clearly liked to stick out, but there was something about the lot of us that meant mischief, and at last he struck. The next thing was to get the money; and where do you think he carried us but to that place with the door?-whipped out a key, went in, and presently came back with the matter of ten pounds in gold and a cheque for the balance on Coutts's, drawn payable to bearer, and signed with a name that I can't mention, though it's one of the points of my story, but it was a name at least very well known and often printed. The figure was stiff; but the signature was good for more than that, if it was only genuine. I took the liberty of pointing out to my gentleman that the whole business looked apocryphal; and that a man does not, in real life, walk into a cellar door at four in the morning and come out of it with another man's cheque for close upon a hundred pounds. But he was quite easy and sneering. 'Set your mind at rest,' says he; 'I will stay with you till the banks open, and cash the cheque myself.' So we all set off, the doctor, and the child's father, and our friend and myself, and passed the rest of the night in my chambers; and next day, when we had breakfasted, went in a body to the bank. I gave in the cheque myself, and said I had every reason to believe it was a forgery. Not a bit of it. The cheque was genuine."

"Tut-tut!" said Mr. Utterson.

"I see you feel as I do," said Mr. Enfield. "Yes, it's a bad story. For my man was a fellow that nobody could have to do with, a really damnable man; and the person that drew the cheque is the very pink of the proprieties, celebrated too, and (what makes it worse) one of your fellows who do what they call good."

Visits to Dr. Jekyll

Robert Louis Stevenson

It was late in the afternoon when Mr. Utterson found his way to Dr. Jekyll's door, where he was at once admitted by Poole, and carried down by the kitchen offices and across a yard which had once been a garden, to the building which was indifferently known as the laboratory or the dissecting-rooms. The doctor had bought the house from the heirs of a celebrated surgeon; and his own tastes being rather chemical than anatomical, had changed the destination of the block at the bottom of the garden. It was the first time that the lawyer had been received in that part of his friend's quarters; and he eyed the dingy windowless structure with curiosity, and gazed round with a distasteful sense of strangeness as he crossed the theatre, once crowded with eager students and now lying gaunt and silent, the tables laden with chemical apparatus, the floor strewn with crates and littered with packing straw, and the light falling dimly through the foggy cupola. At the further end, a flight of stairs mounted to a door covered with red baize; and through this Mr. Utterson was at last received into the doctor's cabinet. It was a large room, fitted round with glass presses, furnished, among other things, with a cheval-glass and a business table, and looking out upon the court by three dusty windows barred with iron. The fire burned in the grate; a lamp was set lighted on the chimney-shelf, for even in the houses the fog began to lie

From Robert Louis Stevenson, *Dr. Jekyll and Mr. Hyde* (London: Dent [Everyman], 1962), pp. 22, 39, 40.

thickly, and there, close up to the warmth, sat Dr. Jekyll, looking deadly sick.

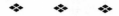

There lay the cabinet before their eyes in the quiet lamplight, a good fire glowing and chattering on the hearth, the kettle singing its thin strain, a drawer or two open, papers neatly set forth on the business table, and nearer the fire, the things laid out for tea; the quietest room, you would have said, and, but for the glazed presses full of chemicals, the most commonplace that night in London.

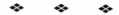

This brought them to the fireside, where the easy chair was drawn cosily up, and the tea things stood ready to the sitter's elbow, the very sugar in the cup. There were several books on a shelf; one lay beside the tea things open, and Utterson was amazed to find it a copy of a pious work for which Jekyll had several times expressed a great esteem, annotated, in his own hand, with startling blasphemies.

Crying Out for the Drug

Robert Louis Stevenson

Mr. Utterson's nerves, at this unlooked-for termination, gave a jerk that nearly threw him from his balance; but he re-collected his courage, and followed the butler into the laboratory building and through the surgical theatre, with its lumber of crates and bottles, to the foot of the stair. Here Poole motioned him to stand on one side and listen; while he himself, setting down the candle and making a great and obvious call on his resolution, mounted the steps, and knocked with a somewhat uncertain hand on the red baize of the cabinet door.

"Mr. Utterson, sir, asking to see you," he called, and even as he did so once more violently signed to the lawyer to give ear.

A voice answered from within: "Tell him I cannot see any one," it said, complainingly.

"Thank you, sir," said Poole, with a note of something like triumph in his voice; and taking up his candle, he led Mr. Utterson back across the yard and into the great kitchen, where the fire was out and the beetles were leaping on the floor.

"Sir," he said, looking Mr. Utterson in the eyes, "was that my master's voice?"

"It seems much changed," replied the lawyer, very pale, but giving look for look.

From Robert Louis Stevenson, *Dr. Jekyll and Mr. Hyde* (London: Dent [Everyman], 1962), pp. 34–36.

"Changed? Well, yes, I think so," said the butler. "Have I been twenty years in this man's house, to be deceived about his voice? No. sir; master's made away with; he was made away with eight days ago, when we heard him cry out upon the name of God; and *who's* in there instead of him, and *why* it stays there, is a thing that cries to Heaven, Mr. Utterson!"

"This is a very strange tale, Poole; this is rather a wild tale, my man," said Mr. Utterson, biting his finger. "Suppose it were as you suppose, supposing Dr. Jekyll to have been—well, murdered, what could induce the murderer to stay? That won't hold water; it doesn't commend itself to reason."

"Well, Mr. Utterson, you are a hard man to satisfy, but I'll do it yet," said Poole. "All this last week (you must know), him, or it, or whatever it is that lives in that cabinet, has been crying night and day for some sort of medicine and cannot get it to his mind. It was sometimes his way— the master's, that is—to write his orders on a sheet of paper and throw it on the stair. We've had nothing else this week back; nothing but papers, and a closed door, and the very meals left there to be smuggled in when nobody was looking. Well, sir, every day, ay, and twice and thrice in the same day, there have been orders and complaints, and I have been sent flying to all the wholesale chemists in town. Every time I brought the stuff back, there would be another paper telling me to return it because it was not pure, and another order to a different firm. This drug is wanted bitter bad, sir, whatever for."

"Have you any of these papers?" asked Mr. Utterson.

Poole felt in his pocket and handed out a crumpled note, which the lawyer, bending nearer to the candle, carefully examined. Its contents ran thus: "Dr. Jekyll presents his compliments to Messrs. Maw. He assures them that their last sample is impure and quite useless for his present purpose. In the year 18—, Dr. J. purchased a somewhat large quantity from Messrs. M. He now begs them to search with the most sedulous care, and should any of the same quality be left, to forward it to him at once. Expense is no consideration. The importance of this to Dr. J. can hardly be exaggerated." So far the letter had run composedly enough; but here, with a sudden splutter of the pen, the writer's emotion had broken loose. "For God's sake," he had added, "find me some of the old."

"This is a strange note," said Mr. Utterson; and then sharply, "How do you come to have it open?"

"The man at Maw's was main angry, sir, and he threw it back to me like so much dirt," returned Poole.

"This is unquestionably the doctor's hand, do you know?" resumed the lawyer.

"I thought it looked like it," said the servant, rather sulkily; and then, with another voice, "But what matters hand of write?" he said. "I've seen him!"

"Seen him?" repeated Mr. Utterson. "Well?"

"That's it!" said Poole. "It was this way. I came suddenly into the theatre from the garden. It seems he had slipped out to look for this drug, or whatever it is; for the cabinet door was open, and there he was at the far end of the room digging among the crates. He looked up when I came in, gave a kind of cry and whipped upstairs into the cabinet. It was but for one minute that I saw him, but the hair stood upon my head like quills. Sir, if that was my master, why had he a mask upon his face? If it was my master, why did he cry out like a rat, and run from me? I have served him long enough. And then . . ." the man paused and passed his hand over his face.

"These are all very strange circumstances," said Mr. Utterson, "but I think I begin to see daylight. Your master, Poole, is plainly seized with one of those maladies that both torture and deform the sufferer, hence, for aught I know, the alteration of his voice; hence the mask and his avoidance of his friends; hence his eagerness to find this drug, by means of which the poor soul retains some hope of ultimate recovery—God grant that he be not deceived! There is my explanation; it is sad enough, Poole, ay, and appalling to consider; but it is plain and natural, hangs well together and delivers us from all exorbitant alarms."

Dr. Jekyll's Experiments

Robert Louis Stevenson

The press marked E was unlocked; and I took out the drawer, had it filled up with straw and tied in a sheet, and returned with it to Cavendish Square.

Here I proceeded to examine its contents. The powders were neatly enough made up, but not with the nicety of the dispensing chemist; so that it was plain they were of Jekyll's private manufacture; and when I opened one of the wrappers, I found what seemed to me a simple crystalline salt of a white colour. The phial, to which I next turned my attention, might have been about half-full of a blood-red liquor, which was highly pungent to the sense of smell, and seemed to me to contain phosphorus and some volatile ether. At the other ingredients I could make no guess. The book was an ordinary version book, and contained little but a series of dates. These covered a period of many years, but I observed that the entries ceased nearly a year ago and quite abruptly. Here and there a brief remark was appended to a date, usually no more than a single word: "double" occurring perhaps six times in a total of several hundred entries; and once very early in the list and followed by several marks of exclamation, "total failure!!!" All this, though it whetted my curiosity, told me little that was definite. Here were a vial of some tincture, a paper of some salt and the record of a series of experiments

From Robert Louis Stevenson, *Dr. Jekyll and Mr. Hyde* (London: Dent [Everyman], 1962), pp. 43–44, 46.

that had led (like too many of Jekyll's investigations) to no end of practical usefulness.

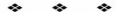

He thanked me with a smiling nod, measured out a few minims of the red tincture and added one of the powders. The mixture, which was at first of a reddish hue, began, in proportion as the crystals melted, to brighten in colour, to effervesce audibly, and to throw off small fumes of vapour. Suddenly, and at the same moment, the ebullition ceased, and the compound changed to a dark purple, which faded again more slowly to a watery green. My visitor, who had watched these metamorphoses with a keen eye, smiled, set down the glass upon the table, and then turned and looked upon me with an air of scrutiny.

Dr. Jekyll's Confession

Robert Louis Stevenson

I was so far in my reflections when, as I have said, a side light began to shine upon the subject from the laboratory table. I began to perceive more deeply than it has ever yet been stated, the trembling immateriality, the mist-like transience, of this seemingly so solid body in which we walk attired. Certain agents I found to have the power to shake and to pluck back that fleshly vestment, even as a wind might toss the curtains of a pavilion. For two good reasons, I will not enter deeply into this scientific branch of my confession. First, because I have been made to learn that doom and burthen of our life is bound for ever on man's shoulders; and when the attempt is made to cast it off, it but returns upon us with more unfamiliar and more awful pressure. Second, because, as my narrative will make, alas! too evident, my discoveries were incomplete. Enough, then, that I not only recognised my natural body for the mere aura and effulgence of certain of the powers that made up my spirit, but managed to compound a drug by which these powers should be dethroned from their supremacy, and a second form and countenance substituted, none the less natural to me because they were the expression, and bore the stamp, of lower elements in my soul.

I hesitated long before I put this theory to the test of practice. I knew well that I risked death; for any drug that so potently controlled

From Robert Louis Stevenson, *Dr. Jekyll and Mr. Hyde* (London: Dent [Everyman], 1962), pp. 49–51, 53, 61–62.

and shook the very fortress of identity, might by the least scruple of an overdose or at the least inopportunity in the moment of exhibition, utterly blot out that immaterial tabernacle which I looked to it to change. But the temptation of a discovery so singular and profound at last overcame the suggestions of alarm. I had long since prepared my tincture; I purchased at once, from a firm of wholesale chemists a large quantity of a particular salt, which I knew, from my experiments, to be the last ingredient required; and, late one night, I compounded the elements, watched them boil and smoke together in the glass and when the ebullition had subsided, with a strong glow of courage, drank off the potion.

The most racking pangs succeeded: a grinding in the bones, deadly nausea that cannot be exceeded at the hour of birth or death. Then these agonies began swiftly to subside, and I came to myself as if out of a great sickness. There was something strange in my sensations, something indescribably new and, from its very novelty, incredibly sweet. I felt younger, lighter, happier in body; within I was conscious of a heady recklessness, a current of disordered sensual images running like a mill race in my fancy, a solution of the bonds of obligation, an unknown but not an innocent freedom of the soul. I knew myself, at the first breath of this new life, to be more wicked, tenfold more wicked, sold a slave to my original evil; and the thought, in that moment, braced and delighted me like wine. I stretched out my hands, exulting in the freshness of these sensations; and in the act, I was suddenly aware that I had lost in stature.

There was no mirror, at that date, in my room; that which stands beside me as I write was brought there later on, and for the very purpose of those transformations. The night, however, was far gone into the morning—the morning, black as it was, was nearly ripe for the conception of the day—the inmates of my house were locked in the most rigorous hours of slumber, and I determined, flushed as I was with hope and triumph, to venture in my new shape as far as to my bedroom. I crossed the yard, wherein the constellations looked down upon me, I could have thought, with wonder, the first creature of that sort that their unsleeping vigilance had yet disclosed to them; I stole through the corridors, a stranger in my own house, and coming to my room, I saw for the first time the appearance of Edward Hyde.

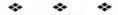

The pleasures which I made haste to seek in my disguise were, as I have said, undignified; I would scarce use a harder term. But in the hands of Edward Hyde they soon began to turn towards the monstrous. When I would come back from these excursions, I was often plunged into a kind of wonder at my vicarious depravity. This familiar that I called out of my own soul, and sent forth alone to do his good pleasure, was a being inherently malign and villainous; his every act and thought centred on self, drinking pleasure with bestial avidity from any degree of torture to another; relentless like a man of stone. Henry Jekyll stood at times aghast before the acts of Edward Hyde; but the situation was apart from ordinary laws, and insidiously relaxed the grasp of conscience. It was Hyde, after all, and Hyde alone, that was guilty. Jekyll was no worse; he woke again to his good qualities seemingly unimpaired; he would even make haste, where it was possible, to undo the evil done by Hyde. And thus his conscience slumbered.

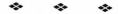

It is useless, and the time awfully fails me, to prolong this description; no one has ever suffered such torments, let that suffice; and yet even to these, habit brought—no, not alleviation—but a certain callousness of soul, a certain acquiescence of despair, and my punishment might have gone on for years, but for the last calamity which has now fallen, and which has finally severed me from my own face and nature. My provision of the salt, which had never been renewed since the date of the first experiment, began to run low. I sent out for a fresh supply, and mixed the drought; the ebullition followed, and the first change of colour, not the second; I drank it, and it was without efficiency. You will learn from Poole how I have had London ransacked; it was in vain; and I am now persuaded that my first supply was impure, and that it was that unknown impurity which lent efficacy to the draught.

About a week has passed, and I am now finishing this statement under the influence of the last of the old powders. This, then, is the last time, short of a miracle, that Henry Jekyll can think his own thoughts or see his own face (now how sadly altered!) in the glass. Nor must I delay too long to bring my writing to an end; for if my narrative has hitherto escaped destruction, it has been by a combination of great prudence and great good luck. Should the throes of change take me in the act of writing it, Hyde will tear it in pieces; but if some time shall have elapsed after I have laid it by, his wonderful selfishness and circumscription to the moment will probably save it once again from the action of his ape-like spite. And indeed the doom that is closing on us both has already changed and crushed him. Half an hour from now when I shall again and for ever reindue that hated personality, I know how I shall sit shuddering and weeping in my chair, or continue, with the most strained and fearstruck ecstasy of listening, to pace up and down this room (my last earthly refuge) and give ear to every sound of menace. Will Hyde die upon the scaffold? or will he find the courage to release himself at the last moment? God knows; I am careless, this is my true hour of death, and what is to follow concerns another than myself. Here, then, as I lay down the pen, and proceed to seal up my confession, I bring the life of that unhappy Henry Jekyll to an end.

7

Advances toward More
Scientific Practice

An Introduction to Selections from
Sinclair Lewis's Arrowsmith

Sinclair Lewis (1885–1951) made his reputation with a series of satirical novels about aspects of American life. In *Main Street* (1920) he took on small town mores, in *Babbitt* (1922) business, and in *Elmer Gantry* (1927) religion. With *Arrowsmith* (1925) it was the turn of medicine. Though awarded a Pulitzer Prize for this work, Lewis turned it down. His reasons for refusing this honor are far from clear; it may be that he was disappointed at not getting it for *Main Street*, which the judges passed over in favor of Edith Wharton's *The Age of Innocence*. In many of his letters he inveighs against the Pulitzer Prize, but he was happy to accept the Nobel Prize for Literature in 1930.

Lewis came from a medical family: his grandfather, father, and uncle were all general practitioners, and he himself as a student thought of following in their footsteps. His brother Claude, a highly respected surgeon in St. Cloud, Minnesota, provided him with information about the world of medicine. Lewis also enlisted the expert advice of the bacteriologist Paul de Kruif, who was fresh from the Rockefeller Institute for Medical Research in New York, and whose *Microbe Hunters* (1926) is still a highly popular history of discoveries in germ theory. After meeting de Kruif in 1922, Lewis spent many hours with him in laboratories where he was instructed about medical scientific matters, particularly the organization and customs in research institutions. De Kruif also helped

155

Lewis to devise convincing professional histories for Arrowsmith and his mentor, the scientist Gottlieb. All these efforts were designed to assure the soundness of the novel's medical context.

The action of *Arrowsmith* spans from 1897 into the 1920s, although no precise dates are cited in its later part. It traces the career of Martin Arrowsmith from his student days in a large Midwestern university, through his years as a family practitioner in the small town, Wheatsylvania, his position as an assistant public health officer in Nautilus, a somewhat larger place in Iowa, his short spell as a pathologist at a fancy clinic in Chicago, and eventually, after he has published an important article in the *Journal of Infectious Diseases*, his promotion to medical researcher at the prestigious McGurk Institute in New York. Through this sequence of situations that Arrowsmith experiences Lewis is able to give a "recapitulation in one man's life of the development of medicine in the United States," as medical historian Charles Rosenberg so aptly wrote in the *American Quarterly* (1963). The gradual transition from older styles of practice to the newer ones that integrate scientific methods is the novel's overarching theme. Arrowsmith's own wavering between his dual attraction to practice and research illustrates both the conflict and the interaction between these twin spheres of medicine.

Doc Vickerson's chaotic office in Elk Mills in the state of Winnemac in 1897 (described in the first selection) is the incarnation of bygone, almost amateurish and certainly unhygienic practice. Flanked by a "foul" waiting-room and the aged widower's unclean bedroom, the "central room was at once business office, consultation room, operating-theater, living-room, poker den, and warehouse for guns and fishing tackle." Primitive medical equipment jostles with the debris of daily existence in a corner where the sink is more often used for washing dishes than for sterilizing instruments. In the jumble of objects discarded on the sink's ledge everything is derelict: "broken," "unlabeled and forgotten," "frayed," and "rusty." The "rusty lancet stuck in a potato" is a vivid emblem of unscientific practice. "The wild raggedness of the room," Lewis comments, "was the soul and symbol of Doc Vickerson." The appellation "Doc" suggests an affectionate familiarity on his patients' part despite his evident scruffiness. But for all his backwardness and slovenliness, one of the two pieces of advice that Doc Vickerson gives to the young Arrowsmith is to "get your basic science"—the other being: "don't be a booze-hoister like me."

Arrowsmith's office in Wheatsylvania in 1910 (described in the second selection) is obviously a vast improvement over Doc Vickerson's, although he has to improvise furnishings with his mother-in-law's and his wife's help because he lacks the capital to buy equipment. He is bombarded with glossy, glamorous catalogues from the New Idea Instrument and Furniture Company offering all sorts of apparatus guaranteed to impress patients, make practice easy, and bring the doctor respect and wealth. The advertising brochures lure doctors into buying machinery with outlandish names ("Panaceatic Electro-Therapeutic Cabinet") with the promise of "honor" and "riches" (see selection 3). "Big fees" as well as respect as "a high-class practitioner" have come to be associated with technological gadgetry. The appeal is to the doctor's materialism and vanity; "Modern Progress" has led to the commercialization of medicine. Here Lewis's satirical streak is strongly to the fore as he indicts the gullibility of patients and the greed of doctors who are both liable to be taken in by spurious contraptions because they look scientific. Lewis indicates the deceptiveness of such claims through the excesses of the catalogue's overblown language and presentation. Nevertheless, indirectly he points to the dangerous exploitation of the idea of "progress" through its perversion into instruments that will bring in revenue. The pursuit of financial reward is a prominent theme throughout the novel from the medical students' conversations to the advice given to Arrowsmith in Nautilus to join a golf and country club as the basis for a lucrative practice, and the ostentatious affluence of Angus Duer, the successful surgeon. Without funds at the start of his career, Arrowsmith makes do with the simplest equipment, turning the former kitchen of his office suite into a laboratory, but he promises his in-laws to concentrate on earning a living and not "to go monkeying with any scientific research."

His first patients bring him satisfaction as well as income. The reference to the telephone is important (see "Telephone and Car," the fourth selection). As early as 1877 the first rudimentary telephone exchange was inaugurated in the Capital Avenue drugstore in Hartford, Connecticut, linked to twenty-one doctors. The telephone call superseded the old slow method of sending for the doctor by a hand-carried note or a verbal message. Another technological innovation that significantly changed medical practice, especially in rural areas, was the advent of the motor car. Since physicians would routinely spend much of their day in making house-calls, the replacement of the horse-and-buggy by a motor vehicle brought a tremendous gain in time, convenience, and income, for with quicker transportation doctors could see more patients and so increase their earnings. Not surprisingly they were among the first to buy automobiles between about 1906 and 1912.

The telephone and the car are pivotal to the incident when Arrowsmith is summoned in the middle of the night to a sick child (see the fifth selection, "A Case of Diphtheria"). Diagnosing diphtheria, he drives forty-eight miles in seventy-nine minutes to fetch the vital antitoxin. A serum to combat diphtheria had been developed in 1894, one of the earliest directly applicable products of laboratory research. But the medication is administered at too advanced a stage in the disease to save the child's life. Dismayed and discouraged, Arrowsmith wonders whether he made the right decision in rushing to fetch the antitoxin. Should he have resorted to the old, sure method of an operation to open up the airpipe? Scientific medicine is shown here as by no means infallible as Arrowsmith faces doubts about the ethical choice he made. Nevertheless, somewhat ironically perhaps, he is praised in a local newspaper report for his courage, enterprise, and scientific skill.

The novel reaches its climax when Arrowsmith goes to a tropical island where there is an outbreak of plague on which he can test the bacteriophage (= bacteria-eater, known just as phage) on which he has been working at the McGurk Institute (see "Plague," the sixth selection). At issue here is the conflict between the long-term benefits to humanity of precisely controlled scientific experimentation and the immediate imperative to succor—and save—suffering, dying people. Gottlieb, the German-born bacteriologist and Arrowsmith's teacher and role model as an impeccable researcher, urges him not to "be just a good doctor" on the island, not to "let anything, not even your own good kind heart, spoil your experiment." By vaccinating half the population and leaving the other half unprotected, Arrowsmith has the ideal opportunity to prove definitively the efficacy of his discovery.

The choice of the plague as the disease on the island endows *Arrowsmith* with a topical dimension. The plague bacillus had been identified in 1894 during an epidemic in Hong Kong by a Japanese bacteriologist, Shibasaburo Kitasato, a pupil of Robert Koch's, and a Swiss microbiologist, Alexandre Yersin out of the Pasteur school. The laboratory played a crucial part in the elaboration of tests to distinguish between different types of plague, but the mechanism whereby the body could acquire immunity against infection was fiercely debated. In 1917 a new theory was proposed by the French-Canadian bacteriologist Félix d'Hérelle (1873–1949) who suggested that a living ultra-microscopic filter-passing virus was responsible for causing the breaking-down of the infective bacteria, thus giving the body immunity against a particular bacterium. He called this virus bacteriophage, signifying one that feeds on living bacteria as a parasite and breaks them down.

Although Arrowsmith is very insistent, before he leaves for the island, on the need for real test cases to prove his experiment, once he arrives there and witnesses the devastation and death caused by the plague, he begins to doubt the legitimacy of pure experimentation. Yet for a while he hardens his heart and sticks to the principles Gottlieb had inculcated into him. Lewis had originally considered *The Shadow of Max Gottlieb* as the title for this novel. Gottlieb, despite his absolute integrity, typifies the intransigent fanaticism of the single-minded researcher. His allegiance is solely to science: it is said that he would prefer to have a patient die of the right treatment than survive by the wrong. Proving beyond any doubt the validity of his findings is of greater importance to him than saving lives in the present because he always privileges the long-term impact of his research. While not at all vicious, like Dr. Griffon in Sue's *Les Mystères de Paris,* Gottlieb reveals the sinister aspects of an exclusive affirmation of science. Arrowsmith feels an obligation to up-hold his mentor's ideals; even when his closest co-worker succumbs, he continues to resist the pressure to give the phage to everyone, proclaiming: "I'm not a sentimentalist; I am a scientist!" However, when he finds his wife dead, he breaks down, drinking heavily, shouting "damn experimentation," and ordering the life-saving phage be given to all who request it. His experiment is ruined. His choice denotes a shortcoming in him as a scientist, but turns him into a warmer figure than Gottlieb, and makes him a more attractive hero for a novel.

Arrowsmith shows the gradual advances toward more scientific practice in the new instrumentation, in public hygiene, in the availability of antitoxin, and above all in bacteriology. But it also dramatizes the growing tensions that problematize progress in the predicaments faced by Arrowsmith himself: the equivocation between laboratory research and medical practice and more fundamentally between his idealism and the rampant commercialization of all aspects of medicine. Even at the McGurk Institute, where scientists are supposed to be free to pursue pure inquiry, Arrowsmith comes up against the covert and later overt push to produce marketable findings. His social reality is fraught with multiple pressures. Because basic laboratory research was slow to produce many immediately usable results, it aroused public exasperation at the mentality typified by Gottlieb. Whereas Lydgate's research project in *Middlemarch* was inspired by idealism and Dr. Jekyll's experimentation in *Dr. Jekyll and Mr. Hyde* largely by sheer curiosity, Arrowsmith's career is repeatedly shaped by the financial considerations that Lewis shows as intrinsic to medicine. But it must not be forgotten that Lewis was above all a social satirist in every sphere.

Ultimately, however, when facing the ethical dilemma about the use of the bacteriophage, Arrowsmith sides with the patients in their demand for prompt healing rather than impeccable science. What are the pros and cons of his choice? Does he merely yield to exhaustion, grief, and guilt at his wife's death? Or does his decision represent a resurgence of his idealism? Is he rebelling against the accepted culture of science? Can this culture be reconciled with his idealism? How are the legitimate imperatives of scientific proof to be weighed against the immediate needs of the mortally sick? Do insufficiently tested new drugs and therapies in the long run pose greater dangers to patients than waiting for conclusive results?

Doc Vickerson's Office

Sinclair Lewis

It was the central room of the three occupied by Doc Vickerson, facing on Main Street above the New York Clothing Bazaar. On one side of it was the foul waiting-room, on the other, the Doc's bedroom. He was an aged widower; for what he called "female fixings" he cared nothing; and the bedroom with its tottering bureau and its cot of frowsy blankets was cleaned only by Martin, in not very frequent attacks of sanitation.

This central room was at once business office, consultation-room, operating-theater, living-room, poker den, and warehouse for guns and fishing tackle. Against a brown plaster wall was a cabinet of zoological collections and medical curiosities, and beside it the most dreadful and fascinating object known to the boy-world of Elk Mills—a skeleton with one gaunt gold tooth. On evenings when the Doc was away, Martin would acquire prestige among the trembling Gang by leading them into the unutterable darkness and scratching a sulfur match on the skeleton's jaw.

On the wall was a home-stuffed pickerel on a home-varnished board. Beside the rusty stove, a sawdust-box cuspidor rested on a slimy oilcloth worn through to the threads. On the senile table was a pile of memoranda of debts which the Doc was always swearing he would "collect from those dead-beats, right now," and which he would never, by any chance, at any time, collect from any of them. A year or two—a decade

From Sinclair Lewis, *Arrowsmith* (New York: Signet Classic, 1961), pp. 6–7.

161

or two—a century or two—they were all the same to the plodding doctor in the bee-murmuring town.

The most unsanitary corner was devoted to the cast-iron sink, which was oftener used for washing eggy breakfast plates than for sterilizing instruments. On its ledge were a broken test-tube, a broken fishhook, an unlabeled and forgotten bottle of pills, a nail-bristling heel, a frayed cigar-butt, and a rusty lancet stuck in a potato.

Arrowsmith's Office in Wheatsylvania

Sinclair Lewis

In the attic Mrs. Tozer found enough seedy chairs for the reception-room, and an ancient bookcase which, when Leora lined it with pink fringed paper, became a noble instrument-cabinet. Till the examining-chair should arrive, Martin would use Wise's lumpy couch, and Leora busily covered it with white oilcloth. Behind the front room of the tiny office-building were two cubicles, formerly bedroom and kitchen. Martin made them into consultation-room and laboratory. Whistling, he sawed out racks for the glassware and turned the oven of a discarded kerosene stove into a hot-air oven for sterilizing glassware.

"But understand, Lee, I'm not going to go monkeying with any scientific research. I'm through with all that."

Leora smiled innocently. While he worked she sat outside in the long wild grass, sniffing the prairie breeze, her hands about her ankles, but every quarter-hour she had to come in and admire.

Mr. Tozer brought home a package at suppertime. The family opened it, babbling. After supper Martin and Leora hastened with the new treasure to the office and nailed it in place. It was a plate-glass sign; on it in gold letters, "M. Arrowsmith, M.D." They looked up, arms about each other, squealing softly, and in reverence he grunted, "There-by-jiminy!"

From Sinclair Lewis, *Arrowsmith* (New York: Signet Classic, 1961), p. 149.

How to Obtain Honor and Riches

Sinclair Lewis

Martin studied the catalogue of the New Idea Instrument and Furniture
Company of New Jersey. It was a handsome thing. On the glossy green
cover, in red and black, were the portraits of the president, a round
quippish man who loved all young physicians; the general manager, a
cadaverous scholarly man who surely gave all his laborious nights and
days to the advancement of science; and the vice-president, Martin's
former preceptor, Dr. Roscoe Geake, who had a lively, eye-glassed, for-
ward-looking modernity all his own. The cover also contained in surprisingly small space, a quantity of poetic prose, and the inspiring promise:

*Doctor, don't be buffaloed by the unenterprising. No reason why YOU
should lack the equipment which impresses patients, makes practice easy, and
brings honor and riches. All the high-class supplies which distinguish the
leaders of the Profession from the Dubs are within YOUR reach right NOW
by the famous New Idea Financial System: "Just a little down and the rest
FREE—out of the increased earnings which New Idea apparatus will bring
you!"*

Above, in a border of laurel wreaths and Ionic capitals, was the
challenge:

*Sing not the glory of soldiers or explorers or statesmen for who can touch
the doctor—wise, heroic, uncontaminated by common greed. Gentlemen, we*

From Sinclair Lewis, *Arrowsmith* (New York: Signet Classic, 1961), pp. 147–148.

164

salute you humbly and herewith offer you the most up-to-the-jiffy catalogue ever presented by any surgical supply house.

The back cover, though it was less glorious with green and red, was equally arousing. It presented illustrations of the Bindlerdorf Tonsillectomy Outfit and of an electric cabinet, with the demand:

Doctor, are you sending your patients off to specialists for tonsil removal or to sanatoriums for electric, etc., treatment? If so, you are losing the chance to show yourself one of the distinguished powers in the domain of medical advancement in your locality, and losing a lot of high fees. Don't you WANT to be a high-class practitioner? Here's the Open Door.

The Bindlerdorf Outfit is not only useful but exquisitely beautiful, adorns and gives class to any office. We guarantee that by the installation of a Bindlerdorf Outfit and a New Idea Panaceatic Electro-Therapeutic Cabinet (see details on pp. 34 and 97) you can increase your income from a thousand to ten thousand annually and please patients more than by the most painstaking plugging.

When the Great call sounds, Doctor, and it's time for you to face your reward, will you be satisfied by a big Masonic funeral and tributes from Grateful Patients if you have failed to lay up provision for the kiddies, and faithful wife who has shared your tribulations?

You may drive through blizzard and August heat, and go down into the purple-shadowed vale of sorrow and wrestle with the ebon-cloaked Powers of Darkness for the lives of your patients, but that heroism is incomplete without Modern Progress, to be obtained by the use of a Bindlerdorf Tonsillectomy Outfit and the New Idea Panaceatic Cabinet, to be obtained on a small payment down, rest on easiest terms known in history of medicine!

Telephone and Car

Sinclair Lewis

Late one afternoon, when he was in a melancholy way preparing to go home, into the office stamped a grizzled Swedish farmer who grumbled, "Doc, I got a fish-hook caught in my thumb and its all swole." To Arrowsmith, intern in Zenith General Hospital with its out-patient clinic treating hundreds a day, the dressing of a hand had been less important than borrowing a match, but to Dr. Arrowsmith of Wheatsylvania it was a hectic operation, and the farmer a person remarkable and very charming. Martin shook his left hand violently and burbled, "Now if there's anything, you just 'phone me—you just 'phone me."

There had been, he felt, a rush of admiring patients sufficient to justify them in the one thing Leora and he longed to do, the thing about which they whispered at night: the purchase of a motor car for his country calls.

They had seen the car at Frazier's store.

It was a Ford, five years old, with torn upholstery, a gummy motor, and springs made by a blacksmith who had never made springs before. Next to the chugging of the gas engine at the creamery, the most familiar sound in Wheatsylvania was Frazier's closing the door of his Ford. He banged it flatly at the store, and usually he had to shut it thrice again before he reached home.

But to Martin and Leora, when they had tremblingly bought the car and three new tires and a horn, it was the most impressive vehicle on earth. It was their own; they could go when and where they wished.

From Sinclair Lewis, *Arrowsmith* (New York: Signet Classic, 1961), p. 150.

A Case of Diphtheria

Sinclair Lewis

So blank, so idle, had been the week that when he heard the telephone at the Tozers', at three in the morning, he rushed to it as though he were awaiting a love message.

A hoarse and shaky voice: "I want to speak to the doctor."

"Yuh—yuh— 'S the doctor speaking."

"This is Henry Novak, four miles northeast, on the Leopolis road. My little girl, Mary, she has a terrible sore throat. I think maybe it is croup and she look awful and—Could you come right away?"

"You bet. Be right there."

Four miles—he would do it in eight minutes.

He dressed swiftly, dragging his worn brown tie together, while Leora beamed over the first night call. He furiously cranked the Ford, banged and clattered past the station and into the wheat prairie. When he had gone six miles by the speedometer, slackening at each rural box to look for the owner's name, he realized that he was lost. He ran into a farm driveway and stopped under the willows, his headlight on a heap of dented milk-cans, broken harvester wheels, cordwood, and bamboo fishing-poles. From the barn dashed a woolly anomalous dog, barking viciously, leaping up at the car.

A frowsy head protruded from a ground-floor window. "What you want?" screamed a Scandinavian voice.

"This is The Doctor. Where does Henry Novak live?"

"Oh! The Doctor! Dr. Hesselink?"

From Sinclair Lewis, *Arrowsmith* (New York: Signet Classic, 1961), pp. 152–156, 157–158.

"No! Dr. Arrowsmith."

"Oh. Dr. Arrowsmith. From Wheatsylvania? Um. Well, you went right near his place. You yoost turn back one mile and turn to the right by the brick schoolhouse, and it's about forty rods up the road—the house with a cement silo. Somebody sick by Henry's?"

"Yuh—yuh—girl's got croup—thanks—"

"Yoost keep to the right. You can't miss it."

Probably no one who has listened to the dire "you can't miss it" has ever failed to miss it.

Martin swung the Ford about, grazing a slashed chopping-block; he rattled up the road, took the corner that side of the schoolhouse instead of this, ran half a mile along a boggy trail between pastures, and stopped at a farmhouse. In the surprising fall of silence, cows were to be heard feeding, and a white horse, startled in the darkness, raised its head to wonder at him. He had to arouse the house with wild squawkings of his horn, and an irate farmer who bellowed, "Who's there? I've got a shot-gun!" sent him back to the country road.

It was forty minutes from the time of the telephone call when he rushed into a furrowed driveway and saw on the doorstep, against the lamplight, a stooped man who called, "The Doctor? This is Novak."

He found the child in a newly finished bedroom of white plastered walls and pale varnished pine. Only an iron bed, a straight chair, a chromo of St. Anne, and a shadeless hand-lamp on a rickety stand broke the staring shininess of the apartment, a recent extension of the farm-house. A heavy-shouldered woman was kneeling by the bed. As she lifted her wet red face, Novak urged:

"Don't cry now; he's here!" And to Martin: "Me little one is pretty bad but we done all we could for her. Last night and tonight we steam her throat, and we put her here in our own bedroom!"

Mary was a child of seven or eight. Martin found her lips and fingertips blue, but in her face no flush. In the effort to expel her breath she writhed into terrifying knots, then coughed up saliva dotted with grayish specks. Martin worried as he took out his clinical thermometer and gave it a professional-looking shake.

It was, he decided, laryngeal croup or diphtheria. Probably diphtheria. No time now for bacteriological examination, for cultures and lei-surely precision. Silva [Arrowsmith's medical school teacher] the healer bulked in the room, crowding out Gottlieb the inhuman perfectionist. Martin leaned nervously over the child on the tousled bed, absent-mindedly trying her pulse again and again. He felt helpless without the equipment of Zenith General, its nurses and Angus Duer's sure advice. He had a sudden respect for the lone country doctor.

He had to make a decision, irrevocable, perhaps perilous. He would use diphtheria antitoxin. But certainly he could not obtain it from Pete Yeska's in Wheatsylvania.

Leopolis?

"Hustle up and get me Blassner, the druggist at Leopolis on the 'phone, he said to Novak, as calmly as he could contrive. He pictured Blassner driving through the night, respectfully bringing the antitoxin to The Doctor. While Novak bellowed into the farm-line telephone in the dining-room, Martin waited—waited—staring at the child; Mrs. Novak waited for him to do miracles; the child's tossing and hoarse gasping became horrible; and the glaring walls, the glaring lines of pale yellow woodwork, hypnotized him into sleepiness. It was too late for anything short of antitoxin or tracheotomy. Should he operate; cut into the windpipe that she might breathe? He stood and worried; he drowned in sleepiness and shook himself awake. He had to do something, with the mother kneeling there, gaping at him, beginning to look doubtful.

"Get some hot cloths—towels, napkins—and keep 'em around her neck. I wish to God he'd get that telephone call!" he fretted.

As Mrs. Novak, padding on thick slippered feet, brought in the hot cloths, Novak appeared with a blank "Nobody sleeping at the drug store, and Blassner's house-line is out of order."

"Then listen. I'm afraid this may be serious. I've got to have antitoxin. Going to drive t' Leopolis and get it. You keep up these hot applications and—Wish we had an atomizer. And room ought to be moister. Got 'n alcohol stove? Keep some water boiling in here. No use of medicine. B' right back."

He drove the twenty-four miles to Leopolis in thirty-seven minutes. Not once did he slow down for a cross-road. He defied the curves, the roots thrusting out into the road, though always one dark spot in his mind feared a blow-out and a swerve. The speeed, the casting away of all caution, wrought in him a high exultation, and it was blessed to be in the cool air and alone, after the strain of Mrs. Novak's watching. In his mind all the while was the page in Osler regarding diphtheria, the very picture of the words: "In severe cases the first dose should be from 8,000—" No. Oh, yes: "—from 10,000 to 15,000 units."

He regained confidence. He thanked the god of science for antitoxin and for the gas motor. It was, he decided, a Race with Death.

"I'm going to do it—going to pull it off and save that poor kid!" he rejoiced.

He approached a grade crossing and hurled toward it, ignoring possible trains. He was aware of a devouring whistle, saw sliding light on the rails, and brought up sharp. Past him, ten feet from his front wheels, flung the Seattle Express like a flying volcano. The fireman was stoking, and even in the thin clearness of coming dawn the glow from the firebox was appalling on the under side of the rolling smoke. Instantly the apparition was gone and Martin sat trembling, hands trembling on the little steering-wheel, foot trembling like St. Vitus's dance on the brake. "That was an awful' close thing!" he muttered, and thought of a widowed Leora, abandoned to Tozers. But the vision of the Novak child, struggling for each terrible breath, overrode all else. "Hell! I've killed the engine!" he groaned. He vaulted over the side, cranked the car, and dashed into Leopolis.

To Crynssen county, Leopolis with its four thousand people was a metropolis, but in the pinched stillness of the dawn it was a tiny graveyard: Main Street a sandy expanse, the low shops desolate as huts. He found one place astir; in the bleak office of the Dakota Hotel the night clerk was playing poker with the 'bus-driver and the town policeman.

They wondered at his hysterical entrance.

"Dr. Arrowsmith, from Wheatsylvania. Kid dying from diphtheria. Where's Blassner live? Jump in my car and show me."

The constable was a lanky old man, his vest swinging open over a collarless shirt, his trousers in folds, his eyes resolute. He guided Martin to the home of the druggist, he kicked the door, then, standing with his lean and bristly visage upraised in the cold early light, he bawled, "Ed! Hey, you, Ed! Come out of it!"

Ed Blassner grumbled from the up-stairs window. To him death and furious doctors had small novelty. While he drew on his trousers and coat he was to be heard discoursing to his drowsy wife on the woes of druggists and the desirability of moving to Los Angeles and going into real estate. But he did have diphtheria antitoxin in his shop, and sixteen minutes after Martin's escape from being killed by a train be was speeding to Henry Novak's.

The child was still alive when he came brusquely into the house.

All the way back he had seen her dead and stiff. He grunted "Thank God!" and angrily called for hot water. He was no longer the embarrassed cub doctor but the wise and heroic physician who had won the Race with Death, and in the peasant eyes of Mrs. Novak, in Henry's nervous obedience he read his power.

Swiftly, smoothly, he made intravenous injection of the antitoxin, and stood expectant.

The child's breathing did not at first vary, as she choked in the labor of expelling her breath. There was a gurgle, a struggle in which her face blackened, and she was still. Martin peered, incredulous. Slowly the

Novaks began to glower, shaky hands at their lips. Slowly they knew the child was gone. In the hospital, death had become indifferent and natural to Martin. He had said to Angus, he had heard nurses say one to another, quite cheerfully, "Well, fifty-seven has just passed out." Now he raged with desire to do the impossible. She *couldn't* be dead. He'd do something—All the while he was groaning, "I should've operated—I should have." So insistent was the thought that for a time he did not realize that Mrs. Novak was clamoring, "She is dead? Dead?"

He nodded, afraid to look at the woman.

"You killed her, with that needle thing! And not even tell us, so we could call the priest!"

He crawled past her lamentations and the man's sorrow and drove home, empty of heart.

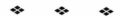

Two weeks after, the *Wheatsylvania Eagle*, a smeary four-page rag, reported:

Our enterprising contemporary, the Leopolis Gazette, *had as follows last week to say of one of our townsmen who we recently welcomed to our midst.*

"Dr. M. Arrowsmith of Wheatsylvania is being congratulated, we are informed by our valued pioneer local physician, Dr. Adam Winter, *by the medical fraternity all through the Pony River Valley, there being no occupation or profession more unselfishly appreciative of each other's virtues than the medical gentlemen, on the courage and enterprise he recently displayed in addition to his scientific skill.*

"Being called to attend the little daughter of Henry Norwalk of near Delft the well-known farmer and finding the little one near death with diphtheria he made a desperate attempt to save it by himself bringing antitoxin from Blassner our ever popular druggist, who had on hand a full and fresh supply. He drove out and back in his gasoline chariot, making the total distance of 48 miles in 79 minutes.

"Fortunately our ever alert policeman, Joe Colby, was on the job and helped Dr. Arrowsmith find Mr. Blassner's bungalow on Red River Avenue and this gentleman rose from bed and hastened to supply the doctor with the needed article but unfortunately the child was already too low to be saved but it is by such incidents of pluck and quick thinking as well as knowledge which make the medical profession one of our greatest blessings."

Plague

Sinclair Lewis

He [Gottlieb] looked perplexed; he peered at Martin as though he did not quite recognize him, and begged:

"Martin, I grow old—not in years—it is a lie I am over seventy—but I have my worries. Do you mind if I give you advice as I have done so often, so many years? Though you are not a schoolboy now in Queen City—no, at Winnemac it was. You are a man and you are a genuine worker. But—

"Be sure you do not let anything, not even your own good kind heart, spoil your experiment at St. Hubert. I do not make funniness about humanitarianism as I used to; sometimes now I t'ink the vulgar and contentious human race may yet have as much grace and good taste as the cats. But if this is to be, there must be knowledge. So many men, Martin, are kind and neighborly; so few have added to knowledge. You have the chance! You may be the man who ends all plague and maybe old Max Gottlieb will have helped, too, *hein,* maybe?

"You must not be just a good doctor at St. Hubert. You must pity, oh, so much the generation after generation yet to come that you can refuse to let yourself indulge in pity for the men you will see dying.

"Dying. . . . It will be peace.

From Sinclair Lewis, *Arrowsmith* (New York: Signet Classic, 1961), pp. 338–339, 358–359, 375–377.

"Let nothing, neither beautiful pity nor fear of your own death, keep you from making this plague experiment complete. And as my friend— If you do this, something will yet have come out of my Directorship. If but one fine thing could come, to justify me—

When Martin came sorrowing into his laboratory he found Terry Wickett waiting.

"Say, Slim," Terry blurted, "just wanted to butt in and suggest, now for St. Gottlieb's sake keep your phage notes complete and up-to-date, and keep 'em in ink!"

"Terry, it looks to me as if you thought I had a fine chance of not coming back with the notes myself."

"Aw, what's biting you!" said Terry feebly.

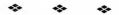

To persuade the shopkeeping lords of St. Hubert to endure a test in which half of them might die, so that all plague might—perhaps—be ended forever, was impossible. Martin argued with Inchcape Jones, with Sondelius, but he had no favor, and he began to meditate a political campaign as he would have meditated an experiment.

He had seen the suffering of the plague and he had (though he still resisted) been tempted to forget experimentation, to give up the possible saving of millions for the immediate saving of thousands. Inchcape Jones, a little rested now under Sondelius's padded bullying and able to slip into a sane routine, drove Martin to the village of Carib, which, because of its pest of infected ground squirrels, was proportionately worse smitten than Blackwater.

They sped out of the capital by white shell roads agonizing to the sun-poisoned eyes; they left the dusty shanties of suburban Yamtown for a land cool with bamboo groves and palmettoes, thick with sugar-cane. From a hilltop they swung down a curving road to a beach where the high surf boomed in limestone caves. It seemed impossible that this joyous shore could be threatened by plague, the slimy creature of dark alleys.

The motor cut through a singing trade wind which told of clean sails and disdainful men. They darted on where the foam feathers below Point Carib and where, round that lone royal palm on the headland, the bright wind hums. They slipped into a hot valley, and came to the village of Carib and to creeping horror.

The plague had been dismaying in Blackwater; in Carib it was the end of all things. The rat-fleas had found fat homes in the ground

squirrels which burrowed in every garden about the village. In Blackwater there had from the first been isolation of the sick, but in Carib death
was in every house, and the village was surrounded by soldier police,
with bayonets, who let no one come or go save the doctors.

Martin was guided down the stinking street of cottages palm-thatched
and walled with cow-dung plaster on bamboo laths, cottages shared by
the roosters and the goats. He heard men shrieking in delirium; a dozen
times he saw that face of terror—sunken bloody eyes, drawn face, open
mouth—which marks the Black Death; and once he beheld an exquisite
girl child in coma on the edge of death, her tongue black and round her
the scent of the tomb.

They fled away, to Point Carib and the trade wind, and when Inchcape
Jones demanded, "After that sort of thing, can you really talk of experimenting?" then Martin shook his head, while he tried to recall the vision
of Gottlieb and all their little plans: "half to get the phage, half to be
sternly deprived."

It came to him that Gottlieb, in his secluded innocence, had not
realized what it meant to gain leave to experiment amid the hysteria of
an epidemic.

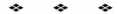

He came up to Penrith Lodge bawling, "Lee! Leora! Come on! *Here* we
are!"

The veranda, as he ran up on it, was leaf-scattered and dusty, and the
front door was banging. His voice echoed in a desperate silence. He was
uneasy. He darted in, found no one in the living-room, the kitchen, then
hastened into their bedroom.

On the bed, across the folds of the torn mosquito netting, was
Leora's body, very frail, quite still. He cried to her, he shook her, he
stood weeping.

He talked to her, his voice a little insane, trying to make her understand that he had loved her and had left her here only for her safety—

There was rum in the kitchen and he went out to gulp down raw
full glasses. They did not affect him.

By evening he strode to the garden, the high and windy garden
looking toward the sea, and dug a deep pit. He lifted her light stiff body,
kissed it, and laid it in the pit. All night he wandered. When he came
back to the house and saw the row of her little dresses with the lines of
her soft body in them, he was terrified.

Then he went to pieces.

He gave up Penrith Lodge, left Twyford's, and moved into a room behind the Surgeon General's office. Beside his cot there was always a bottle.

Because death had for the first time been brought to him, he raged, "Oh, damn experimentation!" and, despite Stokes's dismay, he gave the phage to everyone who asked.

Only in St. Swithin's, since there his experiment was so excellently begun, did some remnant of honor keep him from distributing the phage universally; but the conduct of this experiment he turned over to Stokes.

Stokes saw that he was a little mad, but only once, when Martin snarled, "What do I care for your science?" did he try to hold Martin to his test.

Stokes himself, with Twyford, carried on the experiment and kept the notes Martin should have kept. By evening, after working fourteen or fifteen hours since dawn, Stokes would hasten to St. Swithin's by motor-cycle—he hated the joggling and the lack of dignity and he found it somewhat dangerous to take curving hill-roads at sixty miles an hour, but this was the quickest way, and till midnight he conferred with Twyford, gave him orders for the next day, arranged his clumsy annotations, and marveled at his grim meekness.

Meantime, all day, Martin injected a line of frightened citizens, in the Surgeon General's office in Blackwater. Stokes begged him at least to turn the work over to another doctor and take what interest he could in St Swithin's, but Martin had a bitter satisfaction in throwing away all his significance in helping to wreck his own purposes.

With a nurse for assistant, he stood in the bare office. File on file of people, black, white, Hindu, stood in an agitated cue a block long, ten deep, waiting dumbly, as for death. They crept up to the nurse beside Martin and in embarrassment exposed their arms, which she scrubbed with soap and water and dabbed with alcohol before passing them on to him. He brusquely pinched up the skin of the upper arm and jabbed it with the needle of the syringe, cursing at them for jerking, never seeing their individual faces. As they left him they fluttered with gratitude— "Oh, may God bless you, Doctor!"—but he did not hear.

Sometimes Stokes was there, looking anxious, particularly when in the queue he saw plantation-hands from St. Swithin's, who were supposed to remain in their parish under strict control, to test the value of the phage. Sometimes Sir Robert Fairlamb came down to beam and gurgle and offer his aid. . . . Lady Fairlamb had been Injected first of all, and next to her a tattered kitchen wench, profuse with Hallelujah's.

After a fortnight when he was tired of the drama, he had four doctors making the injections, while he manufactured phage.

8

Emergency

An Introduction to Mikhail Bulgakov's "The Steel Windpipe"

Mikhail Bulgakov (1891–1940) qualified as a doctor in 1916 but gave up the practice of medicine in 1920 to devote himself to writing. His best-known works are the satirical novella *The Heart of a Dog*, completed in 1925 though published in the Soviet Union only in 1987, and *The Master and Margarita*, completed in 1938 and finally published in a full version in 1973. Bulgakov also authored a number of plays but these, too, were perceived as controversial by the Soviet censor and, like his prose works, banned for years on end.

"The Steel Windpipe" is one of several stories that date from early in Bulgakov's career. They appeared between 1925 and 1927 in two monthlies, *Krasnaya panorama*, a magazine aimed at a general readership, and *Meditsinsky rabotnik*, a journal directed at the medical profession. Bulgakov intended to collect the stories into a volume to be entitled *The Notes of a Young Doctor*; however, he never realized this plan so that the stories for long fell into oblivion. Six of them, including "The Steel Windpipe," appeared in 1966 in Bulgakov's *Collected Prose*; three more were unearthed for their first translation into English in 1975 under the title *A Country Doctor's Notebook*.

These stories are clearly autobiographical in origin, drawing on Bulgakov's own experiences as the sole doctor in a remote rural area in the northwestern part of European Russia where he was drafted immediately after his graduation from medical school. By 1916, in the middle of World War I, there was such a critical shortage of medical resources in Russia that newly qualified doctors were sent to government clinics and country hospitals without the important additional training normally provided by the years of internship and residency. Inexperienced, cut off by poor roads, winter blizzards, and a lack of telephones, as well as handicapped by a shortage of proper equipment and supplies, these fledgling physicians were left to cope as best they could, not merely with a wide range of diseases and emergencies but also with the ignorant, superstitious peasants who were their patients. Their only helpers were midwives and semi-skilled assistants known as *feldshers*. The toll taken by the strain of these primitive conditions and the tremendous burden of responsibility is brought out in the story "Morphine" in which another young doctor in the same situation as Bulgakov breaks down under the pressure, becomes addicted to morphine, and eventually commits suicide.

All the stories are, like "The Steel Windpipe," written as first person narratives. All of them, too, insist on the gloom of the extremely long winters, the terrifying isolation, and the doctor's incessant anxieties about his capacity to handle the crises that suddenly occur at the hospital. Generally the anticipatory fear turns out to be worse than the reality. Many of the cases, despite the doctor's trepidation, have a reasonably good outcome, although some patients are recalcitrant, suspicious, and disobedient of orders, taking their medications as they see fit. Occasionally there is even a glimmer of humor at the expense of the exhausted doctor who fails to recognize something obvious such as a baby's "vanishing eye" when covered by an enormous abscess that bursts and drains spontaneously.

"The Steel Windpipe" is a highly dramatic tale in which a child's life is at stake. When she is brought to the hospital by her mother and grandmother, she is already on the verge of death from diphtheria. The peasant women, with mistaken expectations of the hospital, openly vent their anger at the doctor for not having the curative medicine they had hoped for. The extremely slow dissemination of medical progress is illustrated by the fact that diphtheria antitoxin, one of the earliest signal successes of laboratory research, is still not available in these backwoods over twenty years after its first production in 1894. The only hope of saving the little girl's life is a tracheotomy, that is, the insertion of a steel windpipe into her throat in order to drain the pus choking her. This method of treating diphtheria had been devised in 1885. In having recourse to it, the doctor has to continue to use the nineteenth-century methods of treatment even in the second decade of the twentieth century because he has no access to more modern, better means in that remote location.

The situation is an emergency, for the child will soon suffocate without the surgery. The doctor knows theoretically from textbooks the procedure he has to carry out, but he is frightened because he has never actually seen it, let alone done it himself. Here we see a physician facing a private ethical crisis: to do, and perhaps kill the child through ineptitude, or not to do it, thereby letting her die for sure. Secretly he would prefer to be spared the ordeal of such a radical intervention, yet he acknowledges that he should do it. In addition to his own choice, he has to negotiate the mother's consent. The class and educational disparity between the doctor and the peasant women greatly intensifies the difficulty of explaining the life-saving potential of what seems to them a horrible, disfiguring assault on the child. By being absolutely blunt, peremptory, and imperious in addressing the women, the doctor succeeds in securing the mother's agreement.

But even in this story of an emergency, grimness is tempered by humor and especially irony. The detail that the *feldsher*, who should be the doctor's main assistant, faints is quite comical, although it also indicates the horrendousness of watching the child's throat being slit. The midwife's compliment to the doctor, "You did the operation brilliantly, doctor," has an almost ironic ring, yet it is meant seriously and is in fact true under the circumstances. Still more ironical is the impact of the tracheotomy on the peasants, at least as far as the doctor is concerned: the fame of the operation backfires for him because it results in an overwhelming throng of patients. In a characteristic anticlimax the doctor's sole desire at the close is for sleep.

Bulgakov's story is in counterpoint to Sinclair Lewis's *Arrowsmith* where in a similar situation the young physician opts to fetch the antitoxin from the next town, and arrives too late to save the child. Subsequently he wonders whether he ought to have performed a tracheotomy. The fact that the peasant women in "The Steel Windpipe" do, in their desperation, finally bring their dying (grand)daughter to the hospital testifies to their underlying faith in scientific medicine. On the other hand, they naively imagine medical treatment as a form of magic, and are appalled at the proposed surgery. Significantly, the mother, i.e., the younger generation, is persuaded to consent to the procedure while the grandmother, i.e., the older generation, persists in holding out against it. The doctor has to contend not only with the lack of proper supplies and his own inexperience and trepidation but also with a resistant social reality.

"The Steel Windpipe" gives a brilliant evocation of conditions in Russia at the time as well as of the young doctor's thoughts, feelings, and fear of the awful responsibility imposed on him. The extensive use of dialogue creates a sense of urgency and immediacy, while the concision and restraint of the narration throws the spotlight onto the intensity of the protagonists' emotions. As readers we are made to experience vicarious participation in the drama being enacted. Is the doctor's brusqueness toward the child's mother and grandmother justified, or does he go too far toward rudeness? Do his own hesitations diminish his stature, or do they make him heroic in overcoming them?

"The Steel Windpipe"

Mikhail Bulgakov

So I was alone, surrounded by November gloom and whirling snow; the house was smothered in it and there was a moaning in the chimneys. I had spent all twenty-four years of my life in a huge city and thought that blizzards only howled in novels. It appeared that they howled in real life. The evenings here are unusually long, and I fell to daydreaming, staring at the reflection on the window of the lamp with its dark green shade. I dreamed of the nearest town, thirty-two miles away. I longed to leave my country clinic and go there. They had electricity, and there were four doctors whom I could consult. At all events it would be less frightening than this place. But there was no chance of running away, and at times I realised that it would be cowardly. It was for precisely this, after all, that I had been studying medicine.

'Yes, but suppose they bring me a woman in labour and there are complications? Or, say, a patient with a strangulated hernia? What shall I do then? Kindly tell me that. Forty-eight days ago I qualified "with distinction"; but distinction is one thing and hernia is another. Once I watched a professor operating on a strangulated hernia. He did it, while I sat in the amphitheatre. And I only just managed to survive . . .'

More than once I broke out in a cold sweat down my spine at the thought of hernia. Every evening, as I drank my tea, I would sit in the

Mikhail Bulgakov, "The Murderer" from *A Country Doctor's Notebook*. First published in Great Britain by Collins and the Harvill Press, 1975. Translation © Michael Glenny. Reproduced by permission of the Harvill Press.

same attitude: by my left hand lay all the manuals on obstetrical surgery, on top of them the small edition of Döderlein. To my right were ten different illustrated volumes on operative surgery. I groaned, smoked and drank cold tea without milk.

Once I fell asleep. I remember that night perfectly—it was 29 November, and I was woken by someone banging on the door. Five minutes later I was pulling on my trousers, my eyes glued imploringly to those sacred books on operative surgery. I could hear the creaking of sleigh-runners in the yard—my ears had become unusually sensitive. The case turned out to be, if anything, even more terrifying than a hernia or a transverse foetus. At eleven o'clock that night a little girl was brought to the Muryovo hospital. The nurse said tonelessly to me:

'The little girl's weak, she's dying . . . Would you come over to the hospital, please, doctor . . .'

I remember crossing the yard towards the hospital porch, mesmerised by the flickering light of a kerosene lamp. The lights were on in the surgery, and all my assistants were waiting for me, already dressed in their overalls: the *feldsher* Demyan Lukich, young but very capable, and two experienced midwives, Anna Nikolaevna and Pelagea Ivanovna. Only twenty-four years old, having qualified a mere two months ago, I had been placed in charge of the Muryovo hospital.

The *feldsher* solemnly flung open the door and the mother came in— or rather she seemed to fly in, slithering on her ice-covered felt boots, unmelted snow still on her shawl. In her arms she carried a bundle, from which came a steady hissing, whistling sound. The mother's face was contorted with noiseless weeping. When she had thrown off her sheep-skin coat and shawl and unwrapped the bundle, I saw a little girl of about three years old. For a while the sight of her made me forget operative surgery, my loneliness, the load of useless knowledge acquired at university: it was all completely effaced by the beauty of this baby girl. What can I liken her to? You only see children like that on chocolate boxes— hair curling naturally into big ringlets the colour of ripe rye, enormous dark blue eyes, doll-like cheeks. They used to draw angels like that. But in the depths of her eyes was a strange cloudiness and I recognised it as terror—the child could not breathe. 'She'll be dead in an hour,' I thought with absolute certainty, feeling a sharp twinge of pity for the child.

Her throat was contracting into hollows with each breath, her veins were swollen and her face was turning from pink to a pale lilac. I immediately realised what this colouring meant. I made my first diagnosis, which was not only correct but, more important, was given at the same moment as the midwives' with all their experience: 'The little girl has diphtherial croup. Her throat is already choked with membrane and soon it will be blocked completely.'

'How long has she been ill?' I asked, breaking the tense silence of my assistants.

'Five days now,' the mother answered, staring hard at me with dry eyes.

'Diphtheria,' I said to the *feldsher* through clenched teeth, and turned to the mother:

'Why have you left it so long?'

At that moment I heard a tearful voice behind me:

"Five days, sir, five days!"

I turned round and saw that a round-faced old woman had silently come in. 'I wish these old women didn't exist,' I thought to myself. With an aching presentiment of trouble I said:

'Quiet, woman, you're only in the way,' and repeated to the mother: 'Why have you left it so long? Five days? Hmm?' Suddenly with an automatic movement the mother handed the little girl to the grand-mother and sank to her knees in front of me.

'Give her some medicine,' she said and banged her forehead on the floor. 'I'll kill myself if she dies.'

'Get up at once,' I replied, 'or I won't even talk to you.' The mother stood up quickly with a rustle of her wide skirt, took the baby from the grandmother and started rocking it. The old woman turned to the door-post and began praying, while the little girl continued to breathe with a snake-like hiss. The *feldsher* said:

'That's what they're all like. These people!' And he gave a twitch of his moustache.

'Does that mean she's going to die?' the mother asked, staring at me with what looked like black fury.

'Yes, she'll die,' I said quietly and firmly.

The grandmother picked up the hem of her skirt and wiped her eyes. The mother shouted in an ugly voice:

'Give her something! Help her! Give her some medicine!' I could see what was in store for me and remained firm.

'What medicine can I give her? Go on, you tell me. The little girl is suffocating, her throat is already blocked up. For five days you kept her ten miles away from me. Now what do you want me to do?'

'You're the one who's supposed to know,' the old woman whined by my left shoulder in an affected voice which made me immediately detest her.

'Shut up!' I said to her. I turned to the *feldsher* and ordered the little girl to be taken away. The mother handed her to the midwife and the child started to struggle, evidently trying to cry, but her voice could no longer make itself heard. The mother made a protective move towards her, but we kept her away and I managed to look into the little girl's throat by the light of the pressure-lamp. I had never seen diphtheria before except for mild, forgettable cases. Her throat was full of ragged, pulsating, white substance. The little girl suddenly breathed out and spat in my face, but I was so absorbed that I did not flinch.

'Well now,' I said, astonished at my own calm. 'This is the situation: it's late, and the little girl is dying. Nothing will help her except one thing—an operation.'

I was appalled, wondering why I had said this, but I could not help saying it. The thought flashed through my mind: 'What if she agrees to it?'

'How do you mean?' the mother asked.

'I'll have to cut open her throat near the bottom of her neck and put in a silver pipe so that she can breathe, and then maybe we can save her,' I explained.

The mother looked at me as if I was mad and shielded the little girl from me with her arms, while the old woman started muttering again:

'The idea! Don't you let them cut her open! What—cut her throat?'

'Go away, old woman,' I said to her with hatred. 'Inject the camphor!' I ordered the *feldsher*.

The mother refused to hand over the little girl when she saw the syringe, but we explained to her that there was nothing terrible about it.

'Perhaps that will cure her?' she asked.

'No, it won't cure her at all.'

Then the mother burst into tears.

'Stop it,' I said. I took out my watch, and added: 'I'm giving you five minutes to think it over. If you don't agree in five minutes, I shall refuse to do it.'

'I don't agree!' the mother said sharply.

'No, we won't agree to it,' the grandmother put in. 'It's up to you,' I said in a hollow voice, and thought: 'Well, that's that. It makes it easier for me. I've said my piece and given them a chance. Look how dumb-founded the midwives are. They've refused and I'm saved.' No sooner had I thought this than some other being spoke for me in a voice that was not mine:

'Look, have you gone mad? What do you mean by not agreeing? You're condemning the baby to death. You must consent. Have you no pity?'

'No!' the mother shouted once more.

I thought to myself: 'What am I doing? I shall only kill the child.' But I said:

'Come on, come on—you've got to agree! You must! Look, her nails are already turning blue.'

'No, no!'

'All right, take them to the ward. Let them sit there.'

They were led away down the half-lit passage. I could hear the weeping of the women and the hissing of the little girl. The *feldsher* returned almost at once and said:

'They've agreed!'

I felt my blood run cold, but I said in a clear voice:

'Sterilise a scalpel, scissors, hooks and a probe at once.'

A minute later I was running across the yard, through a swirling, blinding snowstorm. I rushed to my room and, counting the minutes, grabbed a book, leafed through it and found an illustration of a tracheotomy. Everything about it was clear and simple: the throat was laid open and the knife plunged into the windpipe. I started reading the text, but could take none of it in—the words seemed to jump before my eyes. I had never seen a tracheotomy performed. 'Ah well, it's a bit late now,' I said to myself, and looked miserably at the green lamp and the clear illustration. Feeling that I had suddenly been burdened with a most fearful and difficult task, I went back to the hospital, oblivious of the snowstorm.

In the surgery a dim figure in full skirts clung to me and a voice whined:

'Oh, sir, how can you cut a little girl's throat? How can you? She's agreed to it because she's stupid. But you haven't got my permission—no you haven't. I agree to giving her medicine, but I shan't allow her throat to be cut.'

'Get this woman out!' I shouted, and added vehemently: 'You're the stupid one! Yes, you are. And she's the clever one. Anyway, nobody asked you! Get her out of here!'

A midwife took a firm hold of the old woman and pushed her out of the room.

'Ready!' the *feldsher* said suddenly.

We went into the small operating theatre; the shiny instruments, blinding lamplight and oilcloth seemed to belong to another world . . . for the last time I went out to the mother, and the little girl could scarcely be torn from her arms. She just said in a hoarse voice: 'My husband's away in town. When he comes back and finds out what I've done, he'll kill me!'

'Yes, he'll kill her,' the old woman echoed, looking at me in horror. 'Don't let them into the operating theatre!' I ordered.

So we were left in the operating theatre, my assistants, myself, and Lidka, the little girl. She sat naked and pathetic on the table and wept soundlessly. They laid her on the table, strapped her down, washed her throat and painted it with iodine. I picked up the scalpel, still wondering what on earth I was doing. It was very quiet. With the scalpel I made a vertical incision down the swollen white throat. Not one drop of blood emerged. Again I drew the knife along the white strip which protruded between the slit skin. Again not a trace of blood. Slowly, trying to remember the illustrations in my textbooks, I started to part the delicate tissues with the blunt probe. At once dark blood gushed out from the lower end of the wound, flooding it instantly and pouring down her neck. The *feldsher* started to staunch it with swabs but could not stop the flow. Calling to mind everything I had seen at university, I set about clamping the edges of the wound with forceps, but this did no good either.

I went cold and my forehead broke out in a sweat. I bitterly regretted having studied medicine and having landed myself in this wilderness. In angry desperation I jabbed the forceps haphazardly into the region of the wound, snapped them shut and the flow of blood stopped immediately. We swabbed the wound with pieces of gauze; now it faced me clean and absolutely incomprehensible. There was no windpipe anywhere to be seen. This wound of mine was quite unlike any illustration. I spent the next two or three minutes aimlessly poking about in the wound, first with the scalpel and then with the probe, searching for the windpipe. After two minutes of this, I despaired of finding it. 'This is the end,' I thought. 'Why did I ever do this? I needn't have offered to do the operation, and Lidka could have died in the ward. As it is she will die with her throat slit open and I can never prove that she would have died anyway, that I couldn't have made it any worse . . .' The midwife wiped my brow in silence. 'I ought to put down my scalpel and say: I don't know what to do next.' As I thought this I pictured the mother's eyes. I picked up the knife again and made a deep, undirected slash into Lidka's neck. The tissues parted and to my surprise the windpipe appeared before me.

'Hooks!' I croaked hoarsely.

The *feldsher* handed them to me. I pierced each side with a hook and handed one of them to him. Now I could see one thing only: the grayish ringlets of the windpipe. I thrust the sharp knife into it—and froze in horror. The windpipe was coming out of the incision and the *feldsher* appeared to have taken leave of his wits: he was tearing it out. Behind me the two midwives gasped. I looked up and saw what was the matter: the *feldsher* had fainted from the oppressive heat and, still holding the hook, was tearing at the windpipe. 'It's fate,' I thought, 'everything's against me. We've certainly murdered Lidka now.' And I added grimly to *myself*: 'As soon as I get back to my room, I'll shoot myself.' Then the older midwife, who was evidently very experienced, pounced on the *feldsher* and tore the hook out of his hand, saying through her clenched teeth:

'Go on, doctor . . .'

The *feldsher* collapsed to the floor with a crash but we did not turn to look at him. I plunged the scalpel into the trachea and then inserted a silver tube. It slid in easily but Lidka remained motionless. The air did not flow into her windpipe as it should have done. I sighed deeply and stopped: I had done all I could. I felt like begging someone's forgiveness for having been so thoughtless as to study medicine. Silence reigned. I could see Lidka turning blue. I was just about to give up and weep, when the child suddenly gave a violent convulsion, expelled a fountain of disgusting clotted matter through the tube, and the air whistled into her windpipe. As she started to breathe, the little girl began to howl. That instant the *feldsher* got to his feet, pale and sweaty, looked at her throat in stupefied horror and helped me to sew it up.

Dazed, my vision blurred by a film of sweat, I saw the happy faces of the midwives and one of them said to me:

'You did the operation brilliantly, doctor.'

I thought she was making fun of me and glowered at her. Then the doors were opened and a gust of fresh air blew in. Lidka was carried out wrapped in a sheet and at once the mother appeared in the doorway. Her eyes had the look of a wild beast. She asked me:

'Well?'

When I heard the sound of her voice, I felt a cold sweat run down my back as I realised what it would have been like if Lidka had died on the table. But I answered her in a very calm voice:

'Don't worry, she's alive. And she'll stay alive, I hope. Only she won't be able to talk until we take the pipe out, so don't let that upset you.'

Just then the grandmother seemed to materialise from nowhere and crossed herself, bowing to the doorhandle, to me, and to the ceiling. This time I did not lose my temper with her, I turned away and ordered Lidka to be given a camphor injection and for the staff to take turns at watching her. Then I went across the yard to my quarters. I remember the green lamp burning in my study, Döderlein lying there and books scattered everywhere. I walked over to the couch fully dressed, lay down and was immediately lost to the world in a dreamless sleep.

A month passed, then another. I grew more experienced and some of the things I saw were rather more frightening than Lidka's throat, which passed out of my mind. Snow lay all around, and the size of my practice grew daily. Early in the new year, a woman came to my surgery holding by the hand a little girl wrapped in so many layers that she looked as round as a little barrel. The woman's eyes were shining. I took a good look and recognised them.

'Ah, Lidka! How are things?'

'Everything's fine.'

The mother unwound the scarves from Lidka's neck. Though she was shy and resisted I managed to raise her chin and took a look. Her pink neck was marked with a brown vertical scar crossed by two fine stitch marks.

'All's well,' I said. 'You needn't come any more.'

'Thank you, doctor, thank you,' the mother said, and turned to Lidka: 'Say thank you to the gentleman!'

But Lidka had no wish to speak to me.

I never saw her again. Gradually I forgot about her. Meanwhile my practice still grew. The day came when I had a hundred and ten patients. We began at nine in the morning and finished at eight in the evening. Reeling with fatigue, I was taking off my overall when the senior midwife said to me:

'It's the tracheotomy that has brought you all these patients. Do you know what they're saying in the villages? The story goes that when Lidka was ill a steel throat was put into her instead of her own and then sewn up. People go to her village especially to look at her. There's fame for you, doctor. Congratulations.'

'So they think she's living with a steel one now, do they?' I enquired.

'That's right. But you were wonderful, doctor. You did it so coolly, it was marvellous to watch.'

'Hm, well, I never allow myself to worry, you know,' I said, not knowing why. I was too tired even to feel ashamed, so I just looked away. I said goodnight and went home. Snow was falling in large flakes, covering everything, the lantern was lit and my house looked silent, solitary and imposing. As I walked I had only one desire—sleep.

9

Telling the Truth

An Introduction to Selections from Thomas Mann's Buddenbrooks

Thomas Mann (1875–1955) is the preeminent German novelist of his time; with the award of the Nobel Prize for Literature in 1929 for *Buddenbrooks* he achieved world-wide fame.

Medical themes are prominent in his works: for example, cholera in *Death in Venice* (1911), tuberculosis in *The Magic Mountain* (1925), which takes place in a sanatorium, and syphilis and encephalitis in *Dr. Faustus* (1947). Most of the members of the Buddenbrook family are afflicted with health disorders of varying kind and severity: one exhibits hypochondria amounting to hysteria, another has a nervous stomach complaint that is clearly psychosomatic, bad teeth are hereditary, and deaths occur from pneumonia, stroke, and typhoid fever. This rather high incidence of maladies in *Buddenbrooks* can be directly related to the novel's underlying theme, which is summarized in its subtitle, "The Decline of a Family."

Though published in 1900, the novel's action takes place between 1835 and 1875 as it traces four generations of the Buddenbrook family. At the outset they are among the city's business, civic, and social leaders; by the end their firm has been taken over, their splendid house sold, and no male heir survives to carry the name forward. The Buddenbrooks fall victim to broken or unsatisfactory marriages, adherence to dated principles, a growing pessimism, poor investment decisions, and an increasing interest in the arts rather than commerce. According to Mann's somewhat romantic hypothesis, their aestheticism undermines their life force.

This decline in the will to live is illustrated by the two instances of dying in "Pneumonia" and "Stroke" (the second and third selections). Elisabeth Buddenbrook, the stalwart matriarch in the second generation, puts up a long, hard fight against the pneumonia that kills her. Before antibiotics, pneumonia was a dangerous, frequently fatal disease which could be treated only by good nursing and scant palliative measures; it was the strength of the body's innate defenses that determined the outcome. Mann evokes the old lady's ever more alarming symptoms with great accuracy and graphic vividness. Indeed, Elisabeth's protracted agony is a harrowing experience for readers who are cast in the position of surrogate spectators alongside her adult children. Yet the course of her illness and her death at an advanced age are within the norm.

By contrast, her son, Thomas's death a mere five years later at a relatively early age is sudden, unexpected, and dramatic. He is felled in the street, apparently by a stroke, following a difficult tooth extraction. The manner of his death has elements that are both realistic and symbolical. In light of the Buddenbrooks's heavy, cholesterol-laden diet and Thomas's burden of stress in both his business and his family, it is wholly credible that an untimely stroke hits him. Symbolism is implicit in his public loss of dignity as his always extremely immaculate clothing is sullied by the slush and mud into which he falls. Unlike his mother, who fights to the very end, Thomas has lost the will to live; hollowed out by his years of effort to keep up appearances, he collapses at a slight provocation and readily succumbs. His demise is established by the application of a stethoscope, an instrument that had not been in use at the time of his mother's illness; the doctors only watch her closely and take her pulse. This detail again shows the slow infiltration of new instruments even in high-class practice.

But despite their disparity, these two deaths also have many fundamental similarities. In both cases the patients are cared for at home, not in hospital, in keeping with the customs of the upper class in the nineteenth century. A private-duty nurse from a religious order is brought into the house. The continuity of traditions is underscored by the appearance of the same Sister Leander.

Even more striking is the constancy of attendance by the same physicians throughout the novel's forty-year time-span. The literary device of the repetition of a motif such as the recurrent description of Dr. Grabow's face as "kindly," "long," and "gentle" also serves to underscore continuity through the sameness. At the beginning of *Buddenbrooks* in "Indigestion" (the first selection), Dr. Grabow looks after little Christian who has upset his stomach by overeating at a family celebration. As in Trollope's *Dr. Thorne* (chapter 2), the family physician is also a family friend who is invited on the festive occasion of the consecration of a new house. Later Thomas discussses political and economic questions with him on a footing of social equality. The same Dr. Grabow, now accompanied by his younger partner, Dr. Langhals, attends Elisabeth in her pneumonia. The seriousness of the case is indicated by their joint visits so as to consult with each other as to the appropriate steps to be taken. By the time of Thomas's death, Dr. Langhals does most of the visiting, but the aged Dr. Grabow also comes to assess the patient's condition.

The underlying issue in all these three cases is that of truth-telling. How much, and when, should the physician divulge to the patient's family, particularly in potentially fatal situations? Even in the very minor disturbance of little Christian's indigestion, Dr. Grabow's ruminations reveal his awareness of the long-term dangers of the heavy eating customary in that society. He realizes full well from experience that many of his patients die suddenly and perhaps prematurely as a direct consequence of their lifestyle. At that time (Christian's indigestion occurs at the opening of the novel's action in 1835), preventive medicine was hardly practiced. Of course, nothing was known about such risk factors as high cholesterol levels, elevated blood pressure, or lack of exercise. Dr. Grabow endorses his patients' bad habits by reflecting on his own pleasure at the large meal he has just taken, including the rich dessert when he was already stuffed. He ignores the implications of Christian's excess, merely prescribing a light diet for a few days, as he always does on such occasions. Perhaps the doctor can be exculpated in this instance because of the absence of scientific information to support his experience. Indeed, in the nineteenth century, when tuberculosis was a major threat, corpulence was considered a sign of good health, while slenderness was viewed with a certain suspicion. The entire incident is given a slightly comical twist by the child's petulant declaration that he wants never again to eat at all. It is as though Mann were echoing the physician's evasion of the issue by his deflection of the narrative toward the humorous.

The doctors' strategy of deliberately skirting round the truth becomes most apparent in the account of Elisabeth's dying. Her son understands the very real peril represented by pneumonia in a woman of her age, but when he raises the question point-blank, he is consoled by bland reassurances regarding her strong constitution. As her condition worsens, the doctors aim at every stage to minimize the disturbing developments. For instance, they suggest bringing in a nurse to take the pressure off the family caregivers, not because the patient needs more expert attention. Similarly, the patient's younger son, Christian, is finally sent for, allegedly to cheer her up, not because her life is in jeopardy. Tact is pushed to such extremes as to amount to deceitfulness. The younger doctor is rather more open in even daring to utter the alarming technical term, "pneumonia," whereas the older one consistently cultivates a misleading reticence or a carefully guarded, noncommittal stance. When he lets the word "danger" slip out (perhaps half intentionally?), he immediately retracts it. Perhaps this is a device used to accustom the relatives gradually to the likelihood of a bad outcome. Yet it suggests the complicated duality of the role he is playing: always maintaining a positive front, but, as if by mistake, sending out a warning signal at last. Thomas's concealment of the truth from his mother is more natural as an effort to protect and encourage her. In a close-knit community, where keeping up appearances at any cost is the cardinal rule, the denial of truth about sickness and impending death is an extension of the convention of covering up unpleasant matters. Elisabeth herself had done this for most of her life, so she willingly accedes to the doctors' evasiveness as a means to stem her mounting anxiety. The doctors, the patient, and the family are all playing the same collusive game.

However, the dynamics are different as she enters the throes of the death struggle. The doctors refuse palliative medications on the grounds that they may hasten her death, and it is a doctor's duty to preserve life as long as possible. They have only the vaguest memories of the religious and moral reasons they had been taught in medical school for upholding this course of action even in the face of imminent death. They appear inhumane and hypocritical not only in withholding medications to alleviate her pain but in their insistent refutation of her suffering when it is evident to all those present at her bedside. Despite their surface geniality and their long-term relationship with the family, they fall short in a crisis because they have a narrow vision of their profession. The patient's pathetic pleas and the family's wishes are overruled by the authority of medical dicta that clearly result in cruelty. The doctors' need to safeguard their conscience takes precedence over succor of the moribund.

At Thomas's deathbed there is less opportunity for pretense since his condition is hopeless all along. Dr. Langhals, who now has primary charge, indicates the necessity of submitting to "God's will," but he is made to seem concerned above all with the impression he is making as he keeps "his beautiful eyes lowered, not devoid of self-satisfaction." As in this instance, Mann's occasional irony prompts readers' questionings, although there is no open criticism of the physicians' conduct in

Buddenbrooks. Mann was writing about a social reality he knew thoroughly from his own life, and what is more, he presents situations through the eyes of the characters, who accept the norms of their time and place.

In contrast to the benign portrayal of the family doctors, the dentist is exposed to ridicule. His whole setting is tawdry from the sludge color of the door to the pervasive cooking smells and the parrot's intrusive shrieks. His servility to Thomas, an eminent member of the community, only highlights his ineptitude as he labors over the extraction. Although the water in the carafe in the waiting-room smells and tastes of chloroform, no mention is made of the administration of any anesthetic. Almost a quarter of a century after it was introduced in Boston, dental anesthesia is still not given in a major German city. The shortfall between medical progress and social reality is very striking here. Anesthesia would likely have reduced the shock to Thomas's system, and perhaps have averted his death.

Buddenbrooks raises a number of critical ethical issues. How well do the doctors in this novel fulfill their function as "confidential friends"? Are they abusing the trust bestowed on them by long intimacy by giving deceptive verbal comfort instead of telling the truth? Or are they correctly assessing the family's desires by adopting this posture? Does their social relationship with the family interfere with their professionalism? Is their reluctance to tell the truth less an expression of dishonesty than a continuation of the rituals of diplomacy, tact, and silence over unpleasant things that govern this society? How does the physician's commitment to preserve life clash with the obligation to mitigate suffering?

Indigestion (Part 1, chapter 7)

Thomas Mann

Where was Dr. Grabow? Mrs. Buddenbrook rose unobtrusively and left the room, for the seats at the foot of the table occupied by the governess, Dr. Grabow, and Christian were empty, and from the hall outside came sounds rather like a repressed lament. She followed the maid who had just served butter, cheese, and fruit, and indeed out there in the half dark little Christian lay, or rather cowered, on the padded seat that encircled the middle pillar, giving out faint, heartbreaking moans.

"Oh dear, Madam!" said the governess who stood by his side next to the doctor, "little Christian is very bad . . ."

"Mama, I feel sick, *damnably* sick!" Christian whimpered while his round, deep-set eyes wandered restlessly about above his rather large nose. He had uttered the work "damnably" only out of an excess of despair, but his mother said:

"If we use such words, dear God punishes us with even worse sickness."

Dr. Grabow felt his pulse; his kindly face seemed to have become even longer and gentler.

"A spot of indigestion . . . nothing terrible," he consoled Mrs. Buddenbrook. And then he continued in his slow, pedantic, professional tone: "It would be best to put him to bed, give him some herbal tea to

From Thomas Mann, *Buddenbrooks* (Frankfurt: Fischer, 1983), pp. 28–29. Translated by Lilian Furst.

194

make him perspire. And strict diet, Mrs. Buddenbrook. As I said, strict diet. A little pigeon, a little toast . . ."

"I don't want any pigeon," screamed Christian, beside himself. "I don't want ever ever to eat again. I feel sick, damnably sick!" The violent word appeared to bring him relief, such was the passion with which he uttered it.

Dr. Grabow smiled to himself, a reflective, somewhat sad smile. Oh, the young fellow would eat again! He would live like everybody. Like his father, relatives and friends, he would spend his days in a sedentary occupation, and four times a day consume heavy and choice things . . . Well, it was God's will! He, Friedrich Grabow, was not the man to upset the life habits of all these good, prosperous, comfortable merchant families. He would come whenever he was called, would recommend strict diet for a day or two—a little pigeon, a little slice of toast, yes indeed, and with a clear conscience assure them that it was nothing serious this time. Young though he was, he had held the hand of many an upright citizen who had eaten his last piece of smoked meat, his last stuffed turkey, and either suddenly and unexpectedly in his office or after a little suffering in his solid old bed had commended his soul to God. A stroke, it was said, a paralysis, a brusque and unforeseen death—yes indeed, and he, Friedrich Grabow, could have predicted it on all those many occasions when he had been called, when perhaps after dinner a strange little bout of dizziness had occurred. Well, it was God's will! He, Friedrich Grabow, was himself not a man who despised stuffed turkey. That ham today with its shallot sauce was delicious, to hell with it, and then, when they were already breathing hard, the pudding—macaroons, raspberries, and custard, yes indeed. "As I said, Mrs. Buddenbrook, strict diet, a little pigeon—a little toast."

Pneumonia (Part 9, chapter 1)

Thomas Mann

Senator Buddenbrook came out of his mother's bedroom into the breakfast room and shut the door behind the two gentlemen, old Dr. Grabow
and young Dr. Langhals, a member of a local family, who had been
practicing in the city for about a year.

"Gentlemen, may I ask you for a moment," he said, and led them
upstairs, along a corridor, through the columned hall into the main
living-room where a fire had already been lit because of the damp, cold
autumn weather. "You will understand my anxiety—please sit down! Set
my mind to rest if that's at all possible."

"That's hard, my dear Senator," answered Dr. Grabow who had
leaned back comfortably with his chin resting on his collar and the brim
of his hat clutched tightly to his body with both hands, while Dr. Langhals,
a stocky man with dark hair, a pointed beard, beautiful eyes, and a vain
expression, had put his top hat down on the carpet and was staring at
his extraordinarily small, hairy hands. "There is, of course, at this point
no reason for any serious concern; you know, in a patient with your
mother's relatively strong resistance. Believe me, as her longstanding
medical adviser, I know her resistance. Really remarkable for her age, I
must say . . ."

From Thomas Mann, *Buddenbrooks* (Frankfurt: Fischer, 1983), pp. 472–476, 483. Translated by Lilian Furst.

"Yes, precisely at her age," the Senator replied uneasily as he twisted the end of his long mustache.

"I am naturally not saying that your mother will be out for a walk again by tomorrow," Dr. Grabow continued softly. "The patient will not have made that impression on you, dear Senator. There's no denying that the catarrh has taken a turn for the worse in the past twenty-four hours. I don't like the attack of shivering last night, and today there is indeed a little stabbing pain and shortness of breath. Some fever too, insignificant, but nevertheless fever. In short, dear Senator, we must face the troubling fact that the lung is a bit affected . . ."

"Inflammation of the lung?" the Senator asked, looking from one doctor to the other.

"Yes—pneumonia," replied Dr. Langhals with a solemn, proper bow.

"But it's just a slight inflammation of the right lung," the family physician answered, "which we must make every effort to localize."

"So there are grounds for serious concern?" The Senator sat quite still, and looked the doctor straight in the eye.

"Concern? well, we must, as I said, take care to limit the illness, to soothe the cough, get the fever down . . . the quinine will do that. And another thing, dear Senator, don't take fright at single symptoms. If the shortness of breath should increase, if at night perhaps some delirium sets in, or tomorrow there's a little discharge, you know, a reddish-brown discharge, even with some blood . . . All that is absolutely to be expected, absolutely a natural part of the illness, absolutely normal. Please also prepare your sister, our dear honored Mrs. Permaneder, who is directing the nursing with so much devotion. How is she by the way? I quite forgot to inquire how her stomach has been these past few days—"

"As usual, nothing new. The worry about her wellbeing naturally takes a back seat now."

"Of course. Yet it occurs to me that your sister needs rest, especially at night, and Miss Severin can't handle things alone . . . How about getting a nurse in, dear Senator? We have our good Catholic sisters, whom you always support so kindly. The Mother Superior will be glad to be of assistance to you."

"So you think that necessary?"

"It's merely a suggestion. It's so pleasant, the sisters are so invaluable. Their experience and calm has such a soothing effect on the patient—particularly in these illnesses that, as I said, produce a number of disturbing symptoms. So, to repeat: you won't grow anxious, will you, my dear Senator? And we shall see, we shall see . . . We will visit again this evening."

"Certainly," said Dr. Langhals as he picked up his top hat and rose together with his senior colleague. But the Senator remained seated, he was not done yet, he had another question in mind, wanted to try another test.

"Gentlemen," he said, "one more thing. My brother Christian is of a nervous disposition, he can't take much. Do you advise me to tell him of this illness? Get him to come back from Hamburg?"

"He's not in town?"

"No, he's in Hamburg, temporarily, on business, as far as I know."

Dr. Grabow threw a look at his colleague; then he shook the Senator's hand with a smile, and said: "So let's leave him to his business. Why alarm him without need? If there should be any development to make his presence desirable, say to calm the patient or to cheer her up . . . well, there'll still be time, still be time."

While the gentlemen returned through the columned hall and the corridor, stopping for a while at the top of the stairs, they spoke of other matters, about politics, about the impact of the recently ended war.

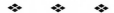

The doctors left, and Senator Buddenbrook turned to go back to the sickroom. He thought over what Dr. Grabow had said. There was so much reticence. You could sense how he shied away from any definite statement. The only unambiguous phrase was "inflammation of the lung" and that became no more reassuring through Dr. Langals's translation into technical language. Inflammation of the lung at his mother's age. The very fact that two doctors were in attendance made the matter more disquieting. Grabow had arranged that quite cannily and almost imperceptibly. He was thinking of retiring sooner or later, he said, and as young Langhals was going to be taking the practice over, so he, Grabow, liked to bring him along now and then so as to introduce him.

When the Senator stepped into the half-darkened sickroom, his expression was cheerful and his bearing energetic. He was so used to concealing worry and fatigue beneath an appearance of secure self-assurance that, as he opened the door, the mask had slipped onto his face almost spontaneously with little effort.

Mrs. Permaneder sat by the four-poster bed, whose curtains were pulled back, and held her mother's hand. The patient, propped up on pillows, turned her head toward her son as he came in, and scrutinized his face searchingly with her light blue eyes. It was a gaze of controlled calm and of intense, inescapable penetration; and coming from the side, it seemed almost stealthy. Apart from the pallor of the skin, which made some feverish spots of redness more visible, her face showed no languor or weakness. The old lady was very alert, more so than those around her for in the last resort she was the one most affected. She distrusted this illness, and was not at all inclined to let go and allow things to take their course.

"What did they say, Thomas?" she asked in such a brisk and lively voice that a violent fit of coughing immediately set in that she tried to suppress by closing her lips, but could not so that she was forced to press her right hand to her side.

"They said," the Senator responded when the bout was over, stroking her hand, "they said that in a few days our good mother would be on her feet again. You can't do it yet, you see, because this stupid cough has naturally attacked the lung a bit . . . it isn't exactly inflammation of the lung," he said, seeing her gaze grow even more penetrating, "although even that wouldn't be the end, there are worse things. In short, the lung is somewhat irritated, they both say, and they may well be right. Where's Miss Severin?"

"Gone to the pharmacy," said Mrs. Permaneder.

"See, there she's gone to the pharmacy again, and you, Tony, look as though you were about to fall asleep at any minute. No, this can't go on. Even if it's only for a few days—we must get a nurse in, don't you agree? I'll ask Mother Superior whether anyone is available."

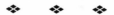

And Sister Leandra came. She put aside her small bag, cape, and the grey bonnet she wore over her white headdress, and with her rosary at her belt making a slight clicking sound, she set to work with soft, friendly words and movements. She nursed the spoiled and at times querulous patient day and night, and then withdrew silently and as if ashamed of the fatigue that overtook her, to go home and sleep a little while another sister took her place.

For the old lady demanded constant attendance at her bedside. The more her condition deteriorated, the more she focused her entire attention, her entire interest on her illness, observing it with fear and an open, naive hatred. Once a woman of the world with a natural ingrained love of the good life, of life itself, she had devoted her last years to piousness and charitable deeds . . . why? Perhaps not only out of loyalty to her deceased husband but also out of the unconscious urge to reconcile heaven to her driving vitality and to induce it to grant her a gentle death despite her former tenacious grasp on life. But she could not die gently. Notwithstanding many painful experiences, her figure had remained completely unbent and her eyes clear. She loved good meals, elegant clothes, ignoring or covering up unpleasant happenings around her, and basking in her elder son's widespread eminence. This illness, this inflammation of the lung had burst in on her erect body without any preliminary psychological preparation to ease its destructiveness . . . that undermining process of suffering that slowly and painfully estranges us from life itself or at least from the conditions under which we have lived, and so arouses in us the sweet longing for an end, for other conditions, for peace. No, she felt that despite her Christian lifestyle of recent years, she was not really ready to die. The thought that, if this were indeed her terminal illness, it must assail her of its own accord, in a final hour and in horrible haste, break her resistance under physical torture and force her surrender: this thought filled her with fear.

She prayed a great deal; but even more, whenever she was conscious, she watched over her condition, felt her pulse, measured her fever, and fought off the cough. But her pulse was bad, the fever rose higher after falling a little, shivers sent her into delirium, the cough and its associated pain and bloody discharge increased, and the shortness of breath frightened her. All this stemmed from the fact that now not merely a segment of the right lung but the whole right lung was affected, indeed it seemed as if the signs of the process were perceptible on the left side too. Dr. Langhals, staring at his nails, called it hepatization, while Dr. Grabow preferred to say nothing. The fever wasted her relentlessly. Her digestion became implicated. Inexorably, slowly, persistently, the decline of her strength progressed.

She followed all this, eagerly ingested the concentrated nutrition offered to her whenever she was able, observed the timing of her medications even more meticulously than the nurses, and was so absorbed in her illness that she spoke almost exclusively with the doctors, or at least showed genuine interest only in conversations with them. Visitors, who were at first allowed, friends, members of her Bible reading group, elderly ladies of her social circle, ministers' wives were received with apathy or distracted cordiality, and quickly dismissed. Family members were embarrassed by the indifference with which the old lady greeted them, a kind of disdain as if to convey: "You can't help me anyway." Even when her small grandson was brought in during a tolerable hour, she only fleetingly stroked his cheek and then turned away. It was as though she wanted to say: "Children, you are all dear people, but I—I must perhaps die!" To both doctors, on the other hand, she extended a lively, warm interest, conferring with them at length.

One day the Gerhardt sisters appeared in their cloaks, their plate-like hats, and their baskets of provisions for visits to the poor, and they would not be put off from seeing their sick friend. They were left alone with her, and heavens only knows what they said as they sat at her bedside. But when they left, their eyes and faces were softer, more radiant, more blissfully remote than ever, and in the sickroom the old lady lay quite still, quite peacefully with the same eyes and expression as they, more peacefully than ever before; her breathing was shallow and at long intervals, and she was clearly declining into greater and greater weakness. Mrs. Permaneder, who sent the Gerhardt ladies off with a murmured strong word, immediately called in the doctors. Both gentlemen had barely appeared at the door when a complete, astonishing change came over the patient. She awoke, she began to move, she nearly sat up. The sight of these two men, these hastily instructed physicians, brought her back to earth abruptly. She stretched out her arms, both arms, toward them, and began: "Welcome, welcome, gentlemen! The situation is this: today, in the course of the day . . ."

But the day had long since come when there was no denying the double inflammation of the lungs.

"Yes, my dear Senator," Dr. Grabow had said, taking Thomas Buddenbrook's hand, "we haven't been able to prevent it, it's now on both sides, and that's always serious, you know that as well as I, I won't beat about the bush. Whether the patient is twenty or seventy, this has to be taken seriously in every case, and if you were to ask me today whether you should write to your brother, Christian, perhaps send him a short telegram, I wouldn't advise you against it, I would think twice about holding you back. How is he, incidentally? A fun fellow, I've always liked him a great deal . . . For heaven's sake, dear Senator, don't draw any exaggerated conclusions from my words. It's not as if there were any immediate danger . . . oh dear, what a fool I am to use such a word! But, you know, under these circumstances one must always look ahead and reckon with unforeseeable occurences. We are quite exceptionally satisfied with your mother as a patient. She is helping us in a stalwart manner, she doesn't let us down . . . no, without paying empty compliments, she is a model patient! And that's why we are hopeful, my dear Senator, hopeful! Let's keep on hoping for the best!"

But there comes a moment when the relatives' hopes have something artificial and inauthentic. A change has already taken place in the patient, an element previously alien to his personality is evident in his behavior. Certain strange words come out of his mouth which we don't know how to counter and which simultaneously cut off his return and oblige him to death. And even if he were our nearest and dearest, beyond this point we can no longer wish him to get up and go his way. Should he nonetheless do so, he would arouse horror like someone who has climbed out of his coffin.

Dreadful signs of the incipient dissolution became apparent while the organs, kept going by a determined will, went on functioning. As several weeks had elapsed since the old lady had had to take to her bed, a number of pressure sores had developed on her body; they would not heal and created a terrible state. She no longer slept, first because of pain, coughing, and shortness of breath, but then also because she herself resisted sleep in order to hang on to wakefulness. Only for minutes did she lose consciousness to fever, but even when fully conscious, she spoke out loud to people who had died long ago. One afternoon in the twilight she said in a loud, somewhat fearful, but fervent voice: "Yes, my dear John, I'm coming!" And the directness of this answer was so compelling that one could almost hear her departed husband's voice calling to her.

Christian arrived; he came from Hamburg where, he reported, he had been on business. He stayed in the sickroom only briefly, then left, wiping his forehead, letting his eyes stray, and saying: "This is terrible, terrible . . . I can't stand any more of it."

Pastor Pringsheim appeared too; he passed Sister Leandra with a cold glance, and prayed at the patient's bedside in a modulated voice.

And then came a brief improvement, an upward turn, a drop in the fever, a deceptive recrudescence of strength, a subsidence of pain, a few clear and hopeful statements, which brought tears to those around the bed.

"We have her, you'll see, we shall keep her despite everything!" said Thomas Buddenbrook. "She'll be with us at Christmas, and we won't let her get as excited as before."

But in the very next night, shortly after Thomas and his wife had gone to bed, they were summoned by Mrs. Permaneder, for the patient was wrestling with death. The wind drove the cold rain that was falling noisily against the window panes.

When the Senator and his wife entered the room, which was lit by candles in two candelabra on the table, both doctors were already there. Christian too had been fetched down from his room and sat somewhere with his back turned to the bed and his head in his hands, bowed down. The patient's brother, who had also been sent for, was expected momentarily. Mrs. Permaneder and her daughter were sobbing silently at the foot of the bed. There was nothing more for Sister Leandra and Miss Severin to do; they looked sadly into the dying woman's face.

She lay on her back, propped up by several pillows, and both her hands, those beautiful blue-veined hands, now so thin and worn, stroked the coverlet with rapid, incessant movements in trembling haste. Her head, covered with a white nightcap, turned restlessly from side to side. Her lips were drawn inward, her mouth opened and closed with a snap at each tortured attempt to breathe, and her sunken eyes roved about as if in search of help; from time to time they rested with a shattering look of envy on one of those present, all of whom were dressed and could breathe, in possession of life and unable to do anything more than make a loving sacrifice that consisted of witnessing her dying. And the night wore on without any change.

"For how long can this go on?" Thomas Buddenbrook asked in a low voice, drawing old Dr. Grabow to the back of the room while Dr. Langhals gave the patient an injection. Mrs. Permaneder, with her hand-kerchief held to her mouth, joined him.

"There's no knowing, dear Senator," Dr. Grabow answered. "Your mother may be released in five minutes, or she could go on living for hours . . . I can't tell. It's a process of suffocation known as edema."

"I understand," said Mrs. Permaneder, nodding into her handker-chief as the tears ran down her cheek. It often happens in inflammation of the lungs . . . A watery liquid accumulates in the lungs' small cells, and when it gets bad, the patient can't breathe . . . Yes, I understand it."

With his hands folded, the Senator looked toward the bed.

"How dreadfully she must be suffering!" he whispered.

"No," said Dr. Grabow in an equally low tone but with immense authority, wrinkling his long, gentle face. "It's deceptive, believe me, dearest friend, it's deceptive. Her consciousness is very clouded. What you see are mostly reflex movements . . . Believe me."

And Thomas replied: "May God grant that it be so!" But any child could see from the old lady's eyes that she was fully conscious, and felt everything.

They sat down again. The old lady's brother had arrived too, and sat at her bedside with red eyes, bent over the handle of his cane.

The patient's movements had increased. A terrible restlessness, an inexpressible fear and distress, an inescapable feeling of abandonment and a boundless helplessness must have permeated this body from the top of her head to the soles of her feet in its condemnation to death. Her eyes, those poor, beseeching, suffering, and imploring eyes sometimes closed with the rattling turns of her head, sometimes opened so wide that the little red blood vessels of the whites stood out bright red. And still no loss of consciousness.

Shortly after three Christian stood up. "I can't take any more," he said, and limped out, leaning on the furniture on the way. Mrs.

Permaneder's daughter and Miss Severin, who had dozed off on their chairs, probably lulled by the rhythmic sounds of pain, looked rosy in their sleep.

At four o'clock it got worse and worse. The patient was propped up, and the sweat wiped off her brow. Her breathing threatened to stop totally, and her panic increased. "Something to make me sleep . . . !" she managed to utter, "a medication!" But there was no intention of giving her anything to make her sleep.

Suddenly she again began to respond to things the others could not hear, as she had done before. "Yes, John, it won't be long!" And immediately afterwards: "Yes, dear Clara, I'm coming!"

And then the struggle was renewed. Was it still a struggle with death? No, now she was struggling with life for death. "I would gladly . . . ," she panted . . . , "I can't . . . Something to make me sleep! Gentlemen, have pity! give me something to make me sleep!"

This "have pity" made Mrs. Permaneder weep out aloud, and Thomas groaned quietly and held his head in his hands. But the doctors knew their duty. It was under all circumstances to preserve this life as long as at all possible for her relatives; a sedative would have caused an immediate, unresisting giving up of the ghost. Doctors' task was not to induce death, but to conserve life at any cost. Besides, this attitude was supported on certain religious and moral grounds, about which they had heard at the university even if they did not have them in mind at the moment. On the contrary, they strengthened her heart with various medications and produced momentary relief by means of retching.

At five the struggle could no longer get any worse. Rising up with wide open eyes, the old lady thrashed her arms as if she were trying to clutch something, or hands that were stretched out toward her, and responded incessantly on every side to calls that she alone heard and that seemed to grow more numerous and insistent. It was as if her parents, her in-laws and several other relatives who had predeceased her were present somewhere. She named names which no one in the room could immediately identify as belonging to specific dead people. "Yes!" she cried, and turned in various directions . . . "Now, I'm coming . . . Right away . . . This very moment. There . . . I can't . . . A medication, gentlemen . . ."

At half past five there was a moment of peace. And then, quite suddenly, her aged face, distorted by suffering, was suffused with a shudder, an abrupt, amazed joy, a profound, quivering, timorous tenderness. With lightning speed she spread out her arms with such trusting and direct rapidity that one felt there was not a second between what she heard and her answer—. With an expression of unconditional obedience and an unlimited yielding and devotion, laden with fear and love, she cried out: "Here I am! . . ." and expired.

They were all scared. What had happened? Who was it that had called to make her follow so immediately?

Someone pulled the drapes back and extinguished the candles, while Dr. Grabow with a gentle expression closed the departed's eyes.

They all shivered in the murky autumn dawn that now filled the room. Sister Leandra covered the dressing table mirror with a cloth.

Stroke (Part 10, chapters 7 and 8)

Thomas Mann

In Mill Street he [Thomas Buddenbrook] entered a house painted in a yellowish-brown color, and mounted to the second floor, where one of the doors bore a brass plate, "Dr. Brecht, Dentist." The corridor was pervaded with a warm smell of beef and cauliflower. Then suddenly he breathed the acrid air of the waiting-room into which he was ushered. "Please take a seat . . . for a moment," the voice of an old woman shrieked out. It was the parrot, Josephus, who sat in a shiny cage at the back of the room and stared at him sidewise mockingly with his venomous little eyes.

The Senator sat down at the round table and tried to savor the jokes in a magazine, but cast it aside in disgust, pressed the cool silver handle of his cane to his cheek, shut his burning eyes, and groaned. It was perfectly quiet except for Josephus who was gnawing and biting at the bars of his cage. Dr. Brecht considered it to be proper, even if he was not engaged, to make his patients wait a while.

Thomas Buddenbrook stood up abruptly and drank a glass of water out of a carafe on the table; it smelled and tasted of chloroform. Then he opened the door onto the corridor, and in an irritated tone shouted to Dr. Brecht to be so good as to hurry up unless he was urgently occupied. He was in pain.

From Thomas Mann, *Buddenbrooks* (Frankfurt: Fischer, 1983), pp. 576–579, 580–581, 582–583. Translated by Lilian Furst.

The dentist's graying mustache, beak nose, and bald head appeared immediately in the door to the operating room.

"Come in, please," he said. "Come in, please!" Josephus too shrieked. The Senator followed without a smile. A difficult case! thought Dr. Brecht, and turned pale.

They both crossed the light room quickly to the big adjustable operating-chair with its padded headrest and green plush velvet armrests that stood in front of one of the two windows. As he sat down, Thomas Buddenbrook explained briefly what was the matter, laid his head back, and shut his eyes.

Dr. Brecht adjusted the chair a little and set to work on the tooth with a tiny mirror and a metal probe. His hand smelled of almond soap, his breath of beef and cauliflower.

"The tooth has to be extracted," he said after a while and turned even paler.

"Go ahead," said the Senator, and shut his eyes even tighter.

Now there was a pause. Dr. Brecht prepared something at a cupboard, and took out some instruments. Then he again came over to the patient.

"I'm going to paint something onto it," he said. And immediately he began to do so, spreading a pungent fluid on the gum. Then quietly and cordially he asked Thomas to sit still and open his mouth wide, and began work.

Thomas Buddenbrook held tight onto the velvet armrests with both hands. He barely felt the forceps being applied and grasping the tooth, but then noticed from the grinding in his mouth as well as from the growing pressure that became more and more violently painful and affected his whole body, that things were well underway. Thank God, he thought. Now it has to take its course. The pain got worse and worse, intolerably agonizing, a veritable catastrophe, rising to an insane, inhuman pitch that tore his brain apart . . . Then it is over; now I must just wait.

It took three or four seconds. Dr. Brecht's quivering exertions were communicated to Thomas Buddenbrook's whole body, he was pulled up slightly in the chair, and heard the soft squeaking sound coming from the dentist's throat . . . Suddenly there was a frightful jerk, a shaking as if his neck were being broken, accompanied by a short cracking, crackling noise. He quickly opened his eyes. The pressure had gone, but his head buzzed, the pain throbbed intensely in the inflamed, damaged jaw, and he sensed clearly that this was not the intended aim, not the true solution to the problem, but a premature catastrophe that only aggravated things. Dr. Brecht had stepped back. He leaned against the instrument cupboard, looking like death, and said:

"The crown . . . That's what I thought."

Thomas Buddenbrook spat out some blood into the blue dish at his side for his gum was injured. Then he asked in semi-consciousness: "What was it you thought? What's up with the crown?"

"The crown has broken, Senator . . . That's what I feared . . . The tooth is in an extraordinarily bad state. But it was my duty to attempt the experiment . . ."

"What next?"

"Leave it to me, Senator . . ."

"What has to be done?"

"The roots have to be removed. By means of a lever . . . There are four of them."

"Four? So four lots of pulling and extracting are necessary?"

"Unfortunately."

"I've had enough for today!" said the Senator, and wanted to get up, yet remained seated and put his head back.

"Dear Sir, one can demand only what is within human limits," he said. "I am not in the best of health . . . I am done in for now. Would you be so good as to open that window for a moment."

Dr. Brecht complied, and then answered: "It's perfectly alright with me, Senator, if you would prefer to come back tomorrow or the day after at a convenient time, and we postpone the operation till then . . . I must admit, I myself . . . I will now take the liberty of rinsing and painting once more in order to reduce the pain temporarily."

He did the rinsing and painting, and then the Senator left, to the accompaniment of the regretful shoulder shrugging into which Mr. Brecht, white as a sheet, put his final strength.

"A moment . . . please!" shrieked Josephus as they went through the waiting-room, and was still shrieking it while Thomas Buddenbrook descended the stairs.

By means of a lever . . . well, that was for tomorrow. What now? Home and rest, try to sleep. The actual pain in the nerve seemed to be numbed, but there was a dull, oppressive burning in his mouth. So, home. And he walked slowly through the streets, mechanically exchanging greetings with those he met; his look was reflective and unsure, as if he were turning over in his mind how he really felt.

He reached his street and began to walk down it along the left sidewalk. After twenty steps he was hit by nausea. I shall have to go into the bar over there and drink a brandy, he thought, and stepped into the road. When he was about halfway across, the following happened to him. It felt exactly as if his brain were being grasped and whirled round with irresistible force at an increasing, terrifyingly increasing speed, first in large, then in ever smaller concentric circles, and finally was shattered with enormous, brutal, pitiless violence against the central stony point of those circles . . . He made a half turn and with arms stretched out in front of him hit the wet pavement.

As the road sloped steeply downhill, the top of his body landed a good deal further down than his feet. He had fallen onto his face, under which a pool of blood immediately began to spread. His hat rolled down the road. His fur coat was spattered with mud and slush. His hands in their white kid gloves were stretched out in a puddle.

He lay like that, and remained there until a few people came and turned him over.

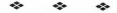

The long flowered curtains stirred in the draught as Mrs. Permaneder, followed by her sister-in-law, entered the bedroom. The smell of carbolic, ether, and other medications wafted toward them. Thomas Buddenbrook lay on his back, undressed, in an embroidered nightgown, under a red coverlet in a broad mahogany bed. His half open eyes were rolled back, under his unkempt mustache his lips moved in a babble as gurgling sounds came now and then out of his throat. Young Dr. Langhals, bent over him, took a blood-soaked bandage off his face, and dipped a clean one in a small bowl on the bedside table. Then he listened to the patient's chest and felt his pulse. At the foot of the bed little Johann sat on a pile of bedclothes, twirled the knot on his sailor suit, listening with a brooding expression to the sounds that came from his father. The soiled clothes hung somewhere on a chair.

Mrs. Permaneder, cowered at the bedside, took hold of her brother's cold, heavy hand, and stared into his face. She began to understand that, whether God knew what he was doing or not, he nevertheless wanted "the worst."

"Tom!" she lamented, "Do you recognize me? How are you? Do you want to leave us? Surely you don't want to leave us? Oh, it *must* not happen . . ."

Nothing that might be taken for an answer ensued. She looked beseechingly up to Dr. Langhals. He stood there, his beautiful eyes lowered, with an expression not devoid of self-satisfaction that reflected God's will.

The governess came in to help with whatever she could. Old Dr. Grabow with his long, gentle face came along personally, shook everyone's

hand, shook his head as he looked at the patient, and did exactly what
Dr. Langhals had already done . . . The news had spread through the
town with lightning speed. The doorbell kept ringing, and inquiries
about the Senator's condition could be heard up in the bedroom. It was
unchanged, unchanged . . . everyone was given the same word.

Both doctors were of the opinion that a nurse must be brought in
for overnight. Sister Leandra was sent for, and she came. There was no
trace of surprise or fear on her face as she entered. This time too she put
down her little leather bag, her bonnet, and her cloak, and set to work
with gentle, friendly movements.

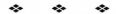

When Dr. Langhals, who had gone home for a while, returned, he found
everything as before. He engaged in a short conversation with the nurse,
and took leave again. Dr. Grabow with his kind face called again too,
checked that everything was being done, and left. Thomas Buddenbrook,
his eyes rolled back, continued to move his lips and emit gurgling sounds.
Evening fell. Faint light from the wintry sunset came in through the
window onto the soiled clothes that hung somewhere over a chair.

At five o'clock Mrs. Permaneder let herself be carried away into an
indiscretion. Sitting with folded hands at the bedside opposite her sister-
in-law, she suddenly began loudly to intone a hymn in her throaty voice:
"Make an end, O Lord," she said, and everyone listened without stir-
ring—"make an end to all his suffering; strengthen his feet and hands,
and let him unto death . . ." But she prayed so fervently from the bottom
of her heart that she kept on concentrating only on the word she was just
saying without realizing that she did not know the end of the verse, and
got stuck ignominiously after the third stanza. She did so, stopped with
her voice raised, and replaced the end with a heightened dignity of
bearing. Everyone in the room waited, and was embarrassed. Little Johann
cleared his throat so strenuously that it sounded like sobbing. And then
in the silence nothing was audible except Thomas Buddenbrook's ago-
nized gurgling.

It was a relief when the maid announced that some food was ready
in the room next door. But as they were beginning to enjoy the soup,
Sister Leandra appeared in the doorway, and nodded to them in a friendly
way.

The Senator was dying. He gulped quietly two or three times, was
silent, and stopped moving his lips. That was the only change that came
over him; his eyes had already been dead before.

Dr. Langhals, who was there a few minutes later, applied his black hearing-rod [stethoscope] to the corpse's chest, listened for a long time, and after conscientious examination pronounced: "Yes, this is the end."

And with the third finger of her pale, gentle hand Sister Leandra carefully shut the dead man's eyelids.

10

A Poor Woman's Plight

An Introduction to Selections from George Moore's Esther Waters

George Moore (1852–1933) was a prolific Anglo-Irish writer who first wrote poetry and then novels about contemporary life. *Esther Waters* (1894), probably his best-known work, was, according to his own account, prompted by Moore's encounter in a London hotel with a maid who aroused his interest in the problems of women servants at the time. The novel was hailed for its candid exposure of the exploitation and wretched working and living conditions of lower class women.

Esther Waters is a good-natured, illiterate young girl who is forced into service in her late teens after her father's death and her mother's remarriage. When two more children are born, her family is unable to support her; her stepfather turns her out of her home so that she has to fend for herself from an early age onward. At first she has a relatively good position in a large household, where her mistress is kind, although the work is hard. But she is dismissed when she becomes pregnant after yielding to the cook's son, whose advances flatter her and with whom she falls in love. Too proud to admit her dilemma, she struggles to cope on her own, getting by on the very scant savings she had managed to accumulate.

One of Esther's major problems is how to get admitted to a hospital for the delivery of her baby. Even if the hospital was not a site for research as in Sue's *Les Mystères de Paris* (chapter 3), it was at that time a source of shame and humiliation as well as of danger to have to resort

213

to a charitable institution. Growing out of almshouses for the indigent, hospitals were a refuge for the poverty-stricken; the middle and upper classes shunned them partly as a social indignity, partly out of a justified fear of cross-infections which were pervasive. Hospitals were seen mainly as places to die for those who had nowhere else to go; those who had homes were looked after there by family and servants. Surgery and certainly births were more safely carried out at home because of the insalubrious conditions in hospitals. Physicians themselves did not favor hospitalization for those who could afford to be cared for in the privacy of their homes. The juxtaposition of *Esther Waters* with Mann's *Buddenbrooks* (chapter 9) illustrates the enormous disparity in the health care available to the have-nots and the haves. By the time of *Esther Waters* attitudes to hospitals had begun to change as they gradually became less life-threatening with the introduction first of antisepsis and then of asepsis (see Introduction). The availability of x-rays in the closing years of the nineteenth century was a decisive inducement to hospital use since the early machines were too cumbersome for a doctor's office, let alone for transport to a home. Private, paying patients were separated in comfortable, better ventilated pavilions from the charity cases. With the rapid advance of ever more complex technology and vastly improved hygiene and nursing, hospitals eventually moved in the twentieth century from the periphery to the very core of medicine as centers for research and the most innovative therapeutics.

In Esther's day hospitals were still primarily charitable institutions funded by benefactors' contributions. In return for their donations regular subscribers had the privilege of a certain number of "letters" per year nominating beneficiaries for admission (see the first selection, "Gaining Admission to Hospital"). The allocation was generally in proportion to the level of the donation so that money played a crucial role in access to health care. Some letters granted hospitalization while others were restricted to outpatient services. Prospective patients had to make the rounds of listed subscribers in order to plead for a "ticket." Esther is handicapped in this search by her inability to read and write, so she has to try to remember the addresses as they are read out to her. She chooses the closest ones in order to save on bus fares. She also has to suffer moralistic censure and the refusal of a "letter" because she is unmarried. After several fruitless attempts, tired out, she abandons her quest, and decides to wait until she is in labor when she will likely be admitted as an emergency.

Once Esther gets into hospital (see the selection, "Giving Birth"), she is frightened by the instruments she sees and the screams she hears.

She wonders whether she will survive childbirth, a realistic concern at the time, as is shown by her mother's death at the birth of her fourth child. She is also disturbed by the medical students' loud laughter and frivolous chatter, which suggest indifference to the patients under their care. On the other hand, they are by no means brutal, as is Dr. Griffon in Sue's *Les Mystères de Paris*, only insensitive and perhaps immature. The entire experience is conveyed through Esther's eyes, ears, and thoughts without any authorial comment from Moore. The homely details about the students' behavior such as their noisy crunching of the candy they are eating and their sudden stampede to a window to look at a passing band are indirect means to make their attitude clear. Esther is pointedly reminded that "they are here to learn," which implies that her function, as a charity case, is to be a useful object for instruction. However, not all the staff are equally callous; one young student and one midwife are gentler and kinder to her. When a qualified doctor is called in because her case is not as simple as expected, he speaks in a low whisper and ushers in "silence and scientific collectedness." Esther is given chloroform, which had first been used in 1847 at the Royal Infirmary in Edinburgh, and gained acceptance as an anesthetic in childbirth after it was twice administered to Queen Victoria. When Esther awakes, her baby has been born, and she is no longer of any interest.

Esther has a positive outcome, for both she and her son survive; yet the episode reveals the continuingly precarious position of the poor patient even in the late-nineteenth-century hospital, utterly powerless teaching (and research) material, at the mercy of benefactors' whims and of medical attendants who may provide the right treatment but who are mostly inconsiderate and uncaring.

On the lowest rung of the social ladder, uneducated, and barely able to earn a subsistence wage for herself, Esther never thinks of questioning the system in which she is captive. She does in fact benefit from medical progress when chloroform is administered to her, but as a charity case she is treated with an indifference amounting to contempt. Since the experience is recounted through her eyes and she simply accepts social reality as it is, there is no open criticism. But the difficulties Esther encounters in getting admitted to a hospital and the treatment given to her once she does get in are bound to raise ethical and practical questions in readers' minds. Is health care a universal human right? Can this right be separated from considerations of cost?

Gaining Admission to Hospital

George Moore

She came at last to an ugly desert place. There was the hospital, square, forbidding; and opposite a tall, lean building with long grey columns. Esther rang, and the great door, some fifteen feet high, was opened by a small boy.

"I want to see the secretary. Is the gentleman in?"

"Yes. Will you come this way?"

She was shown into a waiting-room, and while waiting she looked at the religious prints on the walls. A lad of fifteen or sixteen came in. He said—

"You want to see the secretary?"

"Yes."

"But I'm afraid you can't see him; he's out."

"I have come a long way; is there no one else I can see?"

"Yes, you can see me; I'm his clerk. Have you come to be confined?"

Esther answered that she had.

"But," said the boy, "you are not in labour; we never take any one in before."

"I do not expect to be confined for another month. I came to make arrangements."

"You've got a letter?"

From George Moore, *Esther Waters* (Chicago: Pandora Press, [1977] 1979), pp. 109–111.

"No."

"Then you must get a letter from one of the subscribers."

"But I do not know any."

"You can have a book of their names and addresses."

"But I know no one."

"You needn't know them. You can go and call. Take those that live nearest—that's the way it is done."

"Then will you give me the book?"

"I'll go and get one."

The boy returned a moment after with a small book for which he demanded a shilling. Since she had come to London her hand had never been out of her pocket. She had her money with her; she did not dare leave it at home on account of her father. The clerk looked out the addresses for her and she tried to remember them—two were in Cumberland Place, another was in Bryanstone Square. In Cumberland Place she was received by an elderly lady who said she did not wish to judge any one, but it was her invariable practice to give letters only to married women. There was a delicate smell of perfume in the room; the lady stirred the fire and lay back in her arm-chair. Once or twice Esther tried to withdraw, but the lady, although unswervingly faithful to her principles, seemed not indifferent to Esther's story, and asked her many questions.

"I don't see what interest all that can be to you as you ain't going to give me a letter," Esther answered.

The next house she called at the lady was not at home, but she was expected back presently, and the maidservant asked her to take a seat in the hall. But when Esther refused information about her troubles she was called a stuck-up thing who deserved all she got, and was told there was no use waiting. At the next place she was received by a footman who insisted on her communicating her business to him. Then he said he would see if his master was in. He wasn't in; he must have just gone out. The best time to find him was before half-past ten in the morning.

"He'll be sure to do all he can for you—he always do for the good-looking ones. How did it all happen?"

"What business is that of yours? I don't ask your business."

"Well, you needn't turn that rusty."

At that moment the master entered. He asked Esther to come into his study. He was a tall, youngish-looking man of three or four-and-thirty, with bright eyes and hair, and there was in his voice and manner a kindness that impressed Esther. She wished, however, that she had seen his mother instead of him, for she was more than ever ashamed of her condition. He seemed genuinely sorry for her, and regretted that he had given all his tickets away. Then a thought struck him, and he wrote a letter to one of his friends, a banker in Lincoln's Inn Fields. This gentleman, he said, was a large subscriber to the hospital, and would certainly give her the letter she required.

Giving Birth

George Moore

A week passed away, and then one afternoon, as Esther was sitting alone in her room, there came within her a great and sudden shock: life seemed to be slipping from her, and she sat for some minutes quite unable to move, and all the while a gnawing pain stirred between her shoulders. She knew that her time had come, and when the pain ceased she went downstairs to consult Mrs. Jones.

"Hadn't I better go to the hospital now, Mrs. Jones?"

"Not just yet, my dear; them is but the first labour pains; plenty of time to think of the hospital; we'll see how you are in a couple of hours."

"Will it last so long as that?"

"You'll be lucky if you get it over before midnight. I have been down for longer than that."

"Do you mind my stopping in the kitchen with you? I feel frightened when I'm alone."

"No, I'll be glad of your company. I'll get you some tea presently."

"I could not touch anything. Oh, this is dreadful!" she exclaimed, and she walked to and fro holding her sides, balancing herself dolefully. Often Mrs. Jones stopped in her work about the range and said, looking at her, "I know what it is, I have been through it many a time, we all must, it is our earthly lot." About seven o'clock Esther was clinging to

From George Moore, *Esther Waters* (Chicago: Pandora Press, [1977] 1979), pp. 114–117.

the table, and with pain so vivid on her face that Mrs. Jones laid aside the sausages she was cooking and approached the suffering girl.

"What, is it so bad as all that?"

"Oh," she said, "I think I'm dying, I cannot stand up; give me a chair, give me a chair!" and she sank down upon it, leaning across the table, her face and neck bathed in a cold sweat.

"John will have to get his supper himself; I'll leave these sausages on the hob, and run upstairs and put on my bonnet: the things you intend to bring with you, the baby clothes, are made up in a bundle, aren't they?"

"Yes, yes."

Little Mrs. Jones came running down and threw a shawl over Esther, and it was astonishing what support she lent to the suffering girl, calling on her the whole time to lean on her and not to be afraid. "Now then, dear, you must keep your heart up, we have only a few yards further to go."

"You are too good, you are too kind," Esther said, and she leaned against the wall, and Mrs. Jones rang the bell.

"Keep up your spirits; to-morrow it will be all over. I will come round and see how you are."

The door opened. The porter rang a bell, and a sister came running down.

"Come, come, take my arm," she said, "and breathe hard as you are ascending the stairs." Come along, you mustn't loiter."

On the second landing a door was thrown open, and she found herself in a room full of people, and women.

"What! in there? and all those people?" said Esther.

"Of course, those are the midwives and the students."

She saw that the screams she had heard in the passage proceeded from the bed on the left-hand side. A woman lay there huddled up. And in the midst of her terror Esther was taken behind a screen by the sister who had brought her upstairs and quickly undressed. She was clothed in a chemise a great deal too big for her, and a jacket which was also many sizes too large. She remembered hearing the sister say so at the time. Both windows were wide open, and as she walked across the room she noticed the basins on the floor, the lamp on the round table, and the glint of steel instruments.

The students and the nurses were behind her; she knew they were eating sweets, for she heard a young man ask the young women if they would have any more fondants. Their chatter and laughter jarred on her nerves; but at that moment her pains began again, and she saw the young man whom she had seen handing the sweets approaching her bedside.

"Oh, no, not him, not him!" she cried to the nurse. "Not him, not him! he is too young! Do not let him come near me!"

They laughed loudly, and she buried her head in the pillow, overcome with pain and shame; and when she felt him by her she tried to rise from the bed.

"Let me go! take me away! Oh, you are all beasts!"

"Come, come, no nonsense!" said the nurse; "you can't have what you like, they are here to learn;" and when he had tried the pains she heard the midwife say that it wasn't necessary to send for the doctor. Another said that it would be all over in about three hours' time. "An easy confinement, I should say. The other will be more interesting. . . . " Then they talked of the plays they had seen, and those they wished to see. A discussion arose regarding the merits of a shilling novel which every one was reading, and then Esther heard a stampede of nurses, midwives, and students in the direction of the window. A German band had come into the street.

"Is that the way to leave your patient, sister?" said the student who sat by Esther's bed. A good-looking boy with a fair, plump face. Esther looked into his clear blue, girl-like eyes, wondered, and turned away for shame.

The sister stopped her imitation of a popular comedian, and said, "Oh, she's all right; if they were all like her there'd be very little use our coming here."

"Unfortunately that's just what they are," said another student, a stout little fellow with a pointed red beard, the ends of which caught the light. Esther's eyes often went to those stubble ends, and she hated him for his loud voice and jocularity. One of the midwives, a woman with a long nose and small grey eyes, seemed to mock her, and Esther hoped that this woman would not come near her. She felt that she could not bear her touch. There was something sinister in her face, and Esther was glad when her favourite, a little blonde woman with wavy flaxen hair, came and asked her if she felt better. She looked a little like the young student who still sat by her bedside, and Esther wondered if they were brother and sister, and then she thought that they were sweethearts.

Soon after a bell rang, and the students went down to supper, the nurse in charge promising to warn them if any change should take place. The last pains had so thoroughly exhausted Esther that she had fallen into a doze. But she could hear the chatter of the nurses so clearly that she did not believe herself asleep. And in this film of sleep reality was distorted, and the unsuccessful operation which the nurses were discussing, Esther understood to be a conspiracy against her life. She awoke, listened, and gradually a sense of the truth returned to her. She was in the hospital. . . . The nurses were talking of some one who had died last week. . . . That poor woman in the other bed seemed to suffer dreadful. Would she live through it? Would she herself live to see the morning? How long the time, how fearful the place! . . . If the nurses would only stop talking. . . . The pains would soon begin again. . . . It was awful to lie listening, waiting. The windows were open. The mocking gaiety of the street was borne in on the night wind. Then there came a trampling of feet and sound of voices in the passage-the students and nurses were coming up from supper. At the same moment the pains began to creep up from her knees. One of the young men said that her time had not come. The woman with the sinister look that Esther dreaded, held a contrary opinion. The point was argued, and, interested in the question, the crowd came from the window and collected round the disputants. The young man expounded much medical and anatomical knowledge; the nurses listened with the usual deference of women.

Suddenly the discussion was interrupted by a scream from Esther; it seemed to her that she was being torn asunder, that life was going from her. The nurse ran to her side, a look of triumph came upon her face, and she said, "Now we shall see who's right," and forthwith ran for the doctor. He came running up the stairs; immediately silence and scientific collectedness gathered round Esther. After a brief examination he said, in a low whisper—

"I'm afraid this will not be as easy a case as one might have imagined. I shall administer chloroform."

He placed a small wire case over her mouth and nose, and the sickly odour which she breathed from the cotton wool filled her brain with nausea; it seemed to choke her; life swung before her; at every inhalation she expected to lose sight of the circle of faces.

When she opened her eyes the doctors and nurses were still standing round her, but there was no longer any expression of eager interest on their faces. She wondered at this change, and then out of the silence there came a tiny cry.

"What's that?" Esther asked.

"That's your baby."

"My baby! Let me see it; is it a boy or a girl?"

"It is a boy; it will be given to you when we get you out of the labour ward."

11

Hands-on Medical Training

An Introduction to Selections from
Somerset Maugham's Of Human Bondage

William Somerset Maugham (1874–1965) was himself a qualified physician but chose to be a writer after the success of his first novel, *Liza of Lambeth* (1897) which depicts life in the London slums.

Of Human Bondage (1915) is, together with *The Moon and Sixpence* (1919), regarded as his masterpiece. It draws on some of Maugham's own experiences, especially in its portrayal of medical training, although the novel's hero, Philip, inverts the author's career path by first trying to become an artist in Paris before deciding to follow in his father's footsteps into medicine. Immersion in the demands of medicine is for Philip a welcome relief from the vicissitudes of his long, devastating passion for the fickle Mildred, an escape from the human bondage of his obsessive enthrallment to her.

The second half *Of Human Bondage* shows medical training and hospital work from the student's viewpoint (see the first selection, "The Medical Students"). In contrast to Mann's *Buddenbrooks* (chapter 9) and to Moore's *Esther Waters* (chapter 10), where the medical system is experienced through the eyes of patients, here the angle of vision is predominantly that of physicians. The considerable range of men drawn to medicine is underscored: many from families with a lineage in the profession, some later in life (like Philip) after experimenting in other fields, and some from privileged levels so that they had had a liberal arts education at an ancient university such as Oxford, although this was not a necessary requisite for embarking on medical school. The outcome of their efforts is equally varied: some drop out early on because they do not want to work hard enough; others, after failing the examinations, revert to the lower rank of being pharmacists by qualifying at the "Apothecaries' Hall"; a few will become specialized consultants in Harley Street, London's traditional location for the most distinguished doctors. The account of the medical students already conveys how hierarchical the profession was. There is a wide spectrum not only of ability but also of social and financial background among them. Class distinctions are pronounced and heeded even among students, but there is none of the fascination with money characteristic of the students in Sinclair Lewis's *Arrowsmith* (chapter 7). The course of their careers will exhibit the same range of prestige and status, with some aspiring to the top of the ladder in wealth and standing with a knighthood (the title "Sir"), while others have a hard struggle. No mention is made of women among the medical students.

Philip does not enjoy the basic sciences—anatomy and pathology—that had become the essential foundation of medicine. Medical education changed radically over the course of the nineteenth century. Before medicine turned into a science, medical knowledge was often acquired informally through a two-year apprenticeship to an experienced practitioner. Those seeking to enter the profession lived in their teacher's home, paid him tuition fees, accompanied him on visits to patients, and by watching and imitating learned to assist him as a path to independent practice. In her novel *Wives and Daughters* (1866) Elizabeth Gaskell alludes to the competition to become a pupil of the surgeon, Mr. Gibson, because of his high reputation. The 1858 Medical Registration Act in Great Britain put an end to these haphazard educational arrangements by requiring that all medical practitioners be properly examined and licensed by a central controlling authority, the Conjoint Board of the College of Surgeons and the College of Physicians. When Philip enters medical school in about the mid-1890s, "changes had recently been made in the regulations and the course took five years instead of the four as it had done for those who registered before the autumn of 1892." A little biology and some chemistry were added to the curriculum. The more demanding training resulted in the raising of standards and the selection of better students. Doctors' superior qualifications by the end of the nineteenth century in turn led to a rise in their social status.

While Philip finds the science "very tedious," he enjoys working with patients. "Walking the wards," as it was then called, had been a voluntary and entirely unorganized part of medical education so long as the teaching was primarily theoretical. As late as the 1840s it was left to students to decide on their own curriculum and how to follow it. Walking the wards amounted to little more than looking at the cases and hearing the medical attendants' remarks as they informed students of the patients' progress. But the importance of practical, hands-on contact with patients came increasingly to be recognized and to be incorporated into the training. So walking the wards was converted into a discipline in which the students took the active, not the passive part, working and learning rather than being merely instructed. The emphasis was on the recognition of physical signs as the firm basis for a scientific diagnosis rooted in the analysis of the symptoms. By the late nineteenth century clinical teaching had begun to assume its present predominant place in medical education, and students were questioned in their final examinations on the symptoms, treatment, and complications of various diseases such as scarlet fever, pneumonia, and delirium tremens. These changes in medical training reflect the development of medicine from a theoretical, speculative approach to one better grounded in scientific knowledge.

The scene in an outpatient clinic shows how hospitals were still being run as a philanthropic service to the poor (see the second selection, "The Outpatient Clinic"). "Letters" entitling patients to examination and treatment are distributed at midday to those who have presented themselves rather than given out in advance by donors (see Moore, *Esther Waters*, "Gaining Admission to Hospital"). Dr. Tyrell, the senior physician, still conceives the hospital as "a charitable institution" exclusively for those who cannot afford to pay a doctor. In this view he is somewhat behind the times since patients who were not totally destitute had begun to seek out the expertise available at specialized outpatient clinics. Whether such patients should make payment, or at least partial payment was a matter of lively debate as late as 1900. As Maugham comments: most of the patients "were under the impression that the hospital was an institution of the state, for which they paid out of the rates" (that is, local taxes). They also believed the physicians to be "heavily paid" whereas hospital attendance was a form of unremunerated community service for which doctors expected reward in the respect they gained so that ultimately they would garner more private, paying patients. Nevertheless, the hierarchy in *Of Human Bondage* prefigures that of the modern hospital with Dr. Tyrell as the attending, teaching doctor, the house physicians corresponding to today's residents, and the "clerks" to the medical students.

As in *Les Mystères de Paris* (chapter 3) and in *Esther Waters* (chapter 10), the patients are instructional material, though they are handled rather more humanely. Philip practices bandaging and learns dispensing and auscultation in preparation for his rotations through outpatients, medicine, surgery, and midwifery. Each clerk is charged with performing an examination of a patient and making a tentative diagnosis; his findings and notes are then discussed at length with his fellow-clerks and Dr. Tyrell. Still, the patients are regarded with a certain contempt: the old women, for instance, are "herded along," a term usually applied to animals, yet some of them are quite pleased to be the center of attention. The stethoscope is the vital instrument for examination, applied ritualistically with a dispassionate neutrality except in those cases with "interesting" sounds; then students crowd round eagerly to listen to the chest and so to learn.

Philip excels at interacting with patients, quickly becoming a favorite of theirs on account of his gentleness and capacity for empathy. Because he himself has the handicap of a club foot, he has more understanding of human imperfections than the ruddily healthy, highly successful Dr. Tyrell, who exhibits a "jovial condescension" and "a patronizing air." In his pleasure at his own jokes and in his mischievousness in the writing of complicated prescriprions to "give the dispenser something to do," Dr. Tyrell seems self-centered and arrogant, but he is acknowledged to be a thorough teacher and an astute physician. Philip, by contrast, feels at home with the suffering sick, is able to put them at ease, and to inspire their confidence. He clearly has the qualities of a fine doctor.

Beyond mere cases, obvious or complicated, Philip is aware of the human drama represented by each individual, "life" in all its manifold facets. The sick who present themselves at the outpatient clinic are in many ways revealing of social conditions at the time. As charity cases, they are handled in a demeaning manner, but since they cannot afford to pay for private care, they have no alternative. The harshness of the social system is illustrated in the worker who cannot follow the advice to take lighter work and will likely die prematurely because of the heavy labor he has to do to earn enough to support his family; he accommodates to the realities of the situation with sad resignation. Similarly, the tragedy of tuberulosis among the young is poignantly evoked in the two sisters who know their fate only too well. Yet Maugham also injects an element of black comedy into the scene in the figure of the elderly actress who pretends to be much younger and flirts with the doctor. Although Maugham's novel focuses mainly on the doctors' view, it also gives indirect insight into what it was like to be a patient. In their brief encounters, the patients' responses are as varied as the physicians'.

Of Human Bondage shows the increasing importance of the hospital as a teaching institution and the incorporation of the sciences and of instruments as an accepted part of medical education and practice. In the character of Philip and his patients' response to him, it also emphasizes the necessity for continuing sensitivity to patients as human beings, not merely as examples of diverse pathologies. How essential is a physician's capacity for empathy in his treatment of patients—in other words, the balance of scientific knowledge with human qualities? Is Dr. Tyrell's scoffing attitude toward his patients a product of his high-handed character, or is it portrayed as just the norm within the charity health care system? To what extent does Maugham imply criticism of the prevailing system? Does medical progress in the form of better technology necessarily modify the doctor-patient relationship?

The Medical Students

Somerset Maugham

It is a mixed lot which enters upon the medical profession, and naturally there are some who are lazy and reckless. They think it is an easy life, idle away a couple of years; and then, because their funds come to an end or because angry parents refuse any longer to support them, drift away from the hospital. Others find the examinations too hard for them; one failure after another robs them of their nerve, and, panic-stricken, they forget as soon as they come into the forbidding buildings of the Conjoint Board the knowledge which before they had so pat. They remain year after year, objects of good-humoured scorn to younger men: some of them crawl through the examination of the Apothecaries Hall; others become non-qualified assistants, a precarious position in which they are at the mercy of their employer; their lot is poverty, drunkenness, and Heaven only knows their end. But for the most part medical students are industrious young men of the middle-class with a sufficient allowance to live in the respectable fashion they have been used to; many are the sons of doctors who have already something of the professional manner; their career is mapped out: as soon as they are qualified they propose to apply for a hospital appointment, after holding which (and perhaps a trip to the Far East as a ship's doctor), they will join their father and spend the rest of their days in a country practice. One or two are marked out as excep-

From Somerset Maugham, *Of Human Bondage* (New York: Penguin Books, 1963), pp. 265–267.

tionally brilliant: they will take the various prizes and scholarships which are open each year to the deserving, get one appointment after another at the hospital, go on the staff, take a consulting-room in Harley Street, and, specialising in one subject or another, become prosperous, eminent, and titled.

The medical profession is the only one which a man may enter at any age with some chance of making a living. Among the men of Philip's year were three or four who were past their first youth: one had been in the Navy, from which according to report he had been dismissed for drunkenness; he was a man of thirty, with a red face, a brusque manner, and a loud voice. Another was a married man with two children, who had lost money through a defaulting solicitor [lawyer]; he had a bowed look as if the world were too much for him; he went about his work silently, and it was plain that he found it difficult at his age to commit facts to memory. His mind worked slowly. His effort at application was painful to see.

Philip made himself at home in his tiny rooms. He arranged his books and hung on the walls such pictures and sketches as he possessed. Above him, on the drawing-room floor, lived a fifth-year man called Griffiths; but Philip saw little of him, partly because he was occupied chiefly in the wards and partly because he had been to Oxford. Such of the students as had been to a university kept a good deal together: they used a variety of means natural to the young in order to impress upon the less fortunate a proper sense of their inferiority; the rest of the students found their Olympian serenity rather hard to bear. Griffiths was a tall fellow, with a quantity of curly red hair and blue eyes, a white skin and a very red mouth; he was one of those fortunate people whom everybody liked, for he had high spirits and a constant gaiety. He strummed a little on the piano and sang comic songs with gusto; and evening after evening, while Philip was reading in his solitary room, he heard the shouts and the uproarious laughter of Griffiths' friends above him. He thought of those delightful evenings in Paris where they would sit in the studio, Lawson and he, Flanagan and Clutton, and talk of art and morals, the love-affairs of the present, and the fame of the future. He felt sick at heart. He found that it was easy to make a heroic gesture, but hard to abide by its results. The worst of it was that the work seemed to him very tedious. He had got out of the habit of being asked questions by demonstrators. His attention wandered at lectures. Anatomy was a dreary science, a mere matter of learning by heart an enormous number of facts; dissection bored him; he did not see the use of dissecting out laboriously nerves and arteries when with much less trouble you could see in the diagrams of a book or in the specimens of the pathological museum exactly where they were.

The Outpatient Clinic

Somerset Maugham

At the beginning of the winter session Philip became an out-patients'
clerk. There were three assistant-physicians who took out-patients, two
days a week each, and Philip put his name down for Dr. Tyrell. He was
popular with the students, and there was some competition to be his
clerk. Dr. Tyrell was a tall, thin man of thirty-five, with a very small head,
red hair cut short, and prominent blue eyes: his face was bright scarlet.
He talked well in a pleasant voice, was fond of a little joke, and treated
the world lightly. He was a successful man, with a large consulting practice and a knighthood in prospect. From commerce with students and
poor people he had the patronising air, and from dealing always with the
sick he had the healthy man's jovial condescension, which some consultants achieve as the professional manner. He made the patient feel like a
boy confronted by a jolly schoolmaster; his illness was an absurd piece
of naughtiness which amused rather than irritated.

The student was supposed to attend in the out-patients' room every
day, see cases, and pick up what information he could; but on the days
on which he clerked his duties were a little more definite. At that time
the out-patients' department at St. Luke's consisted of three rooms,
leading into one another, and a large, dark waiting-room with massive
pillars of masonry and long benches. Here the patients waited after
having been given their 'letters' at mid-day; and the long rows of them,

From Somerset Maugham, *Of Human Bondage* (New York: Penguin Books, 1963), pp.
395–402.

bottles and gallipots in hand, some tattered and dirty, others decent enough, sitting in the dimness, men and women of all ages, children, gave one an impression which was weird and horrible. They suggested the grim drawings of Daumier. All the rooms were painted alike, in salmon-colour with a high dado of maroon; and there was in them an odour of disinfectants, mingling as the afternoon wore on with the crude stench of humanity. The first room was the largest and in the middle of it were a table and an office chair for the physician; on each side of this were two smaller tables, a little lower: at one of these sat the house-physician and at the other the clerk who took the 'book' for the day. This was a large volume in which were written down the name, age, sex, profession, of the patient and the diagnosis of his disease.

At half past one the house-physician came in, rang the bell, and told the porter to send in the old patients. There were always a good many of these, and it was necessary to get through as many of them as possible before Dr. Tyrell came at two. The H.P. [house-physician] with whom Philip came in contact was a dapper little man, excessively conscious of his importance: he treated the clerks with condescension and patently resented the familiarity of older students who had been his contemporaries and did not use him with the respect he felt his present position demanded. He set about the cases. A clerk helped him. The patients streamed in. The men came first. Chronic bronchitis, 'a nasty 'acking cough,' was what they chiefly suffered from; one went to the H.P. and the other to the clerk handing in their letters: if they were going on well the words *Rep 14* were written on them, and they went to the dispensary with their bottles or gallipots in order to have medicine given them for fourteen days more. Some old stagers held back so that they might be seen by the physician himself, but they seldom succeeded in this; and only three or four, whose condition seemed to demand his attention, were kept.

Dr. Tyrell came in with quick movements and a breezy manner. He reminded one slightly of a clown leaping into the arena of a circus with the cry: Here we are again. His air seemed to indicate: What's all this nonsense about being ill? I'll soon put that right. He took his seat, asked if there were any old patients for him to see, rapidly passed them in review, looking at them with shrewd eyes as he discussed their symptoms, cracked a joke (at which all the clerks laughed heartily) with the H.P., who laughed heartily too but with an air as if he thought it was rather impudent for the clerks to laugh, remarked that it was a fine day or a hot one, and rang the bell for the porter to show in the new patients.

They came in one by one and walked up to the table at which sat Dr. Tyrell. They were old men and young men and middle-aged men, mostly of the labouring class, dock labourers, draymen, factory hands, barmen;

but some, neatly dressed, were of a station which was obviously superior, shop-assistants, clerks, and the like. Dr. Tyrell looked at these with suspicion. Sometimes they put on shabby clothes in order to pretend they were poor; but he had a keen eye to prevent what he regarded as fraud and sometimes refused to see people who, he thought, could well pay for medical attendance. Women were the worst offenders and they managed the thing more clumsily. They would wear a cloak and a skirt which were almost in rags, and neglect to take the rings off their fingers.

"If you can afford to wear jewellery you can afford a doctor. A hospital is a charitable institution," said Dr. Tyrell.

He handed back the letter and called for the next case.

"But I've got my letter."

"I don't care a hang about your letter; you get out. You've got no business to come and steal the time which is wanted by the really poor." The patient retired sulkily, with an angry scowl.

"She'll probably write a letter to the papers on the gross mismanagement of the London hospitals," said Dr. Tyrell, with a smile, as he took the next paper and gave the patient one of his shrewd glances.

Most of them were under the impression that the hospital was an institution of the state, for which they paid out of the rates, and took the attendance they received as a right they could claim. They imagined the physician who gave them his time was heavily paid.

Dr. Tyrell gave each of his clerks a case to examine. The clerk took the patient into one of the inner rooms; they were smaller, and each had a couch in it covered with black horsehair: he asked his patient a variety of questions, examined his lungs, his heart, and his liver, made notes of fact on the hospital letter, formed in his own mind some idea of the diagnosis, and then waited for Dr. Tyrell to come in. This he did, followed by a small crowd of students, when he had finished the men, and the clerk read out what he had learned. The physician asked him one or two questions, and examined the patient himself. If there was anything interesting to hear students applied their stethoscope: you would see a man with two or three to the chest, and two perhaps to his back, while others waited impatiently to listen. The patient stood among them a little embarrassed, but not altogether displeased to find himself the centre of attention: he listened confusedly while Dr. Tyrell discoursed glibly on the case. Two or three students listened again to recognise the murmur or the crepitation which the physician described, and then the man was told to put on his clothes.

When the various cases had been examined Dr. Tyrell went back into the large room and sat down again at his desk. He asked any student who happened to be standing near him what he would prescribe for a patient he had just seen. The student mentioned one or two drugs.

"Would you?" said Dr. Tyrell. "Well, that's original at all events. I don't think we'll be rash."

This always made the students laugh, and with a twinkle of amusement at his own bright humour the physician prescribed some other drug than that which the student had suggested. When there were two cases of exactly the same sort and the student proposed the treatment which the physician had ordered for the first, Dr. Tyrell exercised considerable ingenuity in thinking of something else. Sometimes, knowing that in the dispensary they were worked off their legs and preferred to give the medicines which they had all ready, the good hospital mixtures which had been found by the experience of years to answer their purpose so well, he amused himself by writing an elaborate prescription.

"We'll give the dispenser something to do. If we go on prescribing *mist: alb:* he'll lose his cunning."

The students laughed, and the doctor gave them a circular glance of enjoyment in his joke. Then he touched the bell and, when the porter poked his head in, said:

"Old women, please."

He leaned back in his chair, chatting with the H.P. while the porter herded along the old patients. They came in, strings of anaemic girls, with large fringes and pallid lips, who could not digest their bad, insufficient food; old ladies, fat and thin, aged prematurely by frequent confinements, with winter coughs; women with this, that, and the other, the matter with them. Dr. Tyrell and his house-physician got through them quickly. Time was getting on, and the air in the small room was growing more sickly. The physician looked at his watch.

"Are there many new women today?" he asked.

"A good few, I think," said the H.P.

"We'd better have them in. You can go on with the old ones."

They entered. With the men the most common ailments were due to the excessive use of alcohol, but with the women they were due to defective nourishment. By about six o'clock they were finished. Philip, exhausted by standing all the time, by the bad air, and by the attention he had given, strolled over with his fellow-clerks to the Medical School to have tea. He found the work of absorbing interest. There was humanity there in the rough, the materials the artist worked on; and Philip felt a curious thrill when it occurred to him that he was in the position of the artist and the patients were like clay in his hands. He remembered with an amused shrug of the shoulders his life in Paris, absorbed in colour, tone, values, Heaven knows what, with the aim of producing beautiful things: the directness of contact with men and women gave a thrill of power which he had never known. He found an endless excitement in looking at their faces and hearing them speak; they came in each with his peculiarity, some shuffling uncouthly, some with a little trip, others with heavy, slow tread, some shyly. Often you could guess their trades by the look of them. You learnt in what way to put your questions so that they should be understood, you discovered on what subjects nearly all lied, and by what inquiries you could extort the truth notwithstanding. You saw the different way people took the same things. The diagnosis of dangerous illness would be accepted by one with a laugh and a joke, by another with dumb despair. Philip found that he was less shy with these people than he had ever been with others; he felt not exactly sympathy, for sympathy suggests condescension; but he felt at home with them. He found that he was able to put them at their ease, and, when he had been given a case to find out what he could about it, it seemed to him that the patient delivered himself into his hands with a peculiar confidence.

"Perhaps," he thought to himself, with a smile, "perhaps I'm cut out to be a doctor. It would be rather a lark if I'd hit upon the one thing I'm fit for."

It seemed to Philip that he alone of the clerks saw the dramatic interest of those afternoons. To the others men and women were only cases, good if they were complicated, tiresome if obvious; they heard murmurs and were astonished at abnormal livers; an unexpected sound in the lungs gave them something to talk about. But to Philip there was much more. He found an interest in just looking at them, in the shape of their heads and their hands, in the look of their eyes and the length of their noses. You saw in that room human nature taken by surprise, and often the mask of custom was torn off rudely, showing you the soul all raw. Sometimes you saw an untaught stoicism which was profoundly moving. Once Philip saw a man, rough and illiterate, told his case was hopeless; and, self-controlled himself, he wondered at the splendid instinct which forced the fellow to keep a stiff upper-lip before strangers. But was it possible for him to be brave when he was by himself, face to face with his soul, or would he then surrender to despair? Sometimes there was tragedy. Once a young woman brought her sister to be examined, a girl of eighteen, with delicate features and large blue eyes, fair hair that sparkled with gold when a ray of autumn sunshine touched it for a moment, and a skin of amazing beauty. The students' eyes went to her with little smiles. They did not often see a pretty girl in these dingy rooms. The elder woman gave the family history, father and mother had died of phthisis [tuberculosis], a brother and a sister, these two were the only ones left. The girl had been coughing lately and losing weight. She took off her blouse and the skin of her neck was like milk. Dr. Tyrell examined her quietly, with his usual rapid method; he told two or three of his clerks to apply their stethoscopes to a place he indicated with his finger; and then she was allowed to dress. The sister was standing a little apart and she spoke to him in a low voice, so that the girl should not hear. Her voice trembled with fear.

"She hasn't got it, doctor, has she?"

"I'm afraid there's no doubt about it."

"She was the last one. When she goes I shan't have anybody."

She began to cry, while the doctor looked at her gravely; he thought she too had the type; she would not make old bones either. The girl turned round and saw her sister's tears. She understood what they meant. The colour fled from her lovely face and tears fell down her cheeks. The two stood for a minute or two, crying silently, and then the older, forgetting the indifferent crowd that watched them, went up to her, took her in her arms, and rocked her gently to and fro as if she were a baby.

When they were gone a student asked:

"How long d'you think she'll last, sir?" Dr. Tyrell shrugged his shoulders.

"Her brother and sister died within three months of the first symptoms. She'll do the same. If they were rich one might do something. You can't tell these people to go to St. Moritz [the Swiss mountains where wealthy tuberculosis patients were sent]. Nothing can be done for them."

Once a man who was strong and in all the power of his manhood came because a persistent aching troubled him and his club [insurance]-doctor did not seem to do him any good; and the verdict for him too was death, not the inevitable death that horrified and yet was tolerable because science was helpless before it, but the death which was inevitable because the man was a little wheel in the great machine of a complex civilization, and had as little power of changing the circumstances as an automaton. Complete rest was his only chance. The physician did not ask impossibilities.

"You ought to get some very much lighter job."

"There ain't no light jobs in my business."

"Well, if you go on like this you'll kill yourself. You're very ill."

"D'you mean to say I'm going to die?"

"I shouldn't like to say that, but you're certainly unfit for hard work."

"If I don't work who's to keep the wife and the kids?"

Dr. Tyrell shrugged his shoulders. The dilemma had been presented to him a hundred times. Time was pressing and there were many patients to be seen.

"Well, I'll give you some medicine and you can come back in a week and tell me how you're getting on."

The man took his letter with the useless prescription written upon it and walked out. The doctor might say what he liked. He did not feel so bad that he could not go on working. He had a good job and he could not afford to throw it away.

"I give him a year," said Dr. Tyrell.

Sometimes there was comedy. Now and then came a flash of cockney humour, now and then some old lady, a character such as Charles Dickens might have drawn, would amuse them by her garrulous oddities. Once a woman came who was a member of the ballet at a famous music-hall. She looked fifty, but gave her age as twenty-eight. She was outrageously painted and ogled the students impudently with large black eyes; her smiles were grossly alluring. She had abundant self-confidence and treated Dr. Tyrell, vastly amused, with the easy familiarity with which she might have used an intoxicated admirer. She had chronic bronchitis, and told him it hindered her in the exercise of her profession.

"I don't know why I should 'ave such a thing, upon my word I don't. I've never 'ad a day's illness in my life. You've only got to look at me to know that."

She rolled her eyes round the young men, with a long sweep of her painted eyelashes, and flashed her yellow teeth at them. She spoke with a cockney accent, but with an affectation of refinement which made every word a feast of fun.

"It's what they call a winter cough," answered Dr. Tyrell gravely. "A great many middle-aged women have it."

"Well, I never! That is a nice thing to say to a lady. No one ever called me middle-aged before."

She opened her eyes very wide and cocked her head on one side, looking at him with indescribable archness.

"That is the disadvantage of our profession," said he. "It forces us sometimes to be ungallant."

She took the prescription and gave him one last, luscious smile.

"You will come and see me dance, dearie, won't you?"

"I will indeed."

He rang the bell for the next case.

"I am glad you gentlemen were here to protect me."

But on the whole the impression was neither of tragedy nor of comedy. There was no describing it. It was manifold and various; there were tears and laughter, happiness and woe; it was tedious and interesting and indifferent; it was as you saw it: it was tumultuous and passionate; it was grave; it was sad and comic; it was trivial; it was simple and complex; joy was there and despair; the love of mothers for their children, and of men for women; lust trailed itself through the rooms with leaden feet, punishing the guilty and the innocent, helpless wives and wretched children; drink seized men and women and cost its inevitable price; death sighed in these rooms; and the beginning of life, filling some poor girl with terror and shame, was diagnosed there. There was neither good nor bad there. There were just facts. It was life.

12

A Woman Doctor?

An Introduction to Selections from
Sarah Orne Jewett's A Country Doctor

Sarah Orne Jewett (1849–1909) was born and lived in Maine, the setting for her narratives. *The Country of the Pointed Firs* (1896) is considered a masterpiece of regional writing.

A Country Doctor (1884), one of her earlier novels, has recently gained
increased attention as a result of the interest in women writers. It is autobiographical in origin: Jewett's father was a country doctor, and she
herself aspired to follow in his footsteps but delicate health following an
accident prevented her from fulfilling this ambition. The novel's titular
figure, Dr. Leslie, is a rather idealized character, clearly modeled on Jewett's
view of her own father, while the young Nan Prince seems a wish projec-
tion on the author's part, able to accomplish what she could not.

A Country Doctor actually portrays two country doctors: at the
beginning, Dr. Leslie, and by the end, Nan too. Dr. Leslie, a widower
who has also lost his only child, lives alone except for his housekeeper,
Marilla. His entire life is devoted to his patients whose personal and
family histories he knows well. Deeply caring, he is repeatedly character-
ized by the adverbs *kindly*, *warmly*, *patiently*, and *compassionately*. These
qualities are illustrated early on in the novel by his visit to Captain Finch,
who suffers from the effects of a bad fall on shipboard years ago and is
confined to a secluded farm. Dr. Leslie goes to him "more from the
courtesy and friendliness of the thing than from any hope of giving
professional assistance" (43). He takes along a handful of his best cigars

239

and a bottle of wine, which will do the patient more good than ordinary medications. There are many similarities between Dr. Leslie and Trollope's Dr. Thorne (chapter 2) in their personal relationships with their patients. Throughout the town and its surroundings Dr. Leslie is "a repository of many secrets; he was a friend who could be trusted always" (93).

Dr. Leslie's great, benign impact is made apparent in the first excerpt ("Enter Dr. Leslie") when he is summoned to a moribund young woman: "the benefaction of his presence was felt by every one" (26). He is gentle and understanding in his handling of Adeline, who has returned home in mysterious circumstances, clutching her baby daughter. This episode forms a dramatic opening to *A Country Doctor* as well as a good introduction to Dr. Leslie.

Late in the century Dr. Leslie still practices an essentially old style of medicine, dependent on shrewd observation, long experience, and knowledge of his patients, both physically and psychologically. He is never portrayed using any instruments, although he makes a trip to Boston to "visit the instrument-makers' shops and some bookstores" (113). In the conversation between Dr. Leslie and Dr. Ferris (in the second selection, "Practical Men versus Theorists"), an old medical school friend, who has traveled widely as a ship's doctor, the value of aptitude, intuition, and practical experience is defended in preference to "all the theories of the hour" (83). This passage is a fine example of the controversies of the time and of the skepticism of older physicians toward innovations. Medical progress is not shown as universally and immediately accepted with enthusiasm.

While Dr. Leslie is the dominant figure in the initial part of the novel, the focus then shifts increasingly onto Nan. She is Adeline's baby daughter, who is brought up by her grandmother. When the old lady feels close to death, she asks Dr. Leslie to become the child's guardian. Again, in a manner somewhat parallel to *Dr. Thorne* (when Sir Roger begs the doctor to look after his son), this trust in the doctor reveals the almost family feeling between doctors and patients. Nan's move into Dr. Leslie's house fosters her curiosity about medicine, especially when she accompanies him on his rounds (see the third selection), becoming his "assistant and attendant" (66). Her initiative in putting splints onto a turkey's broken leg is a vivid episode to show her inventiveness and her gift for healing. It turns out that she has inherited these traits from her father, who had also been a doctor.

Nan's determination to become a doctor is the novel's central topic. *A Country Doctor* is one of a cluster of five American fictions that address this theme from divergent angles in the decade between 1881 and 1891:

Dr. Breen's Practice (1881) by William Dean Howells, *Doctor Zay* (1882) by Elizabeth Stuart Phelps, *The Bostonians* (1886) by Henry James, and *Helen Brent, M.D.* (1891) by Annie Nathan Meyer. These works are clearly expressions of the puzzlement, scandal—and fascination—with the newly emergent social phenomenon of the woman doctor. All are set in the Northeast, which had the highest concentration of women doctors: by 1890, 210 women were practicing in Boston alone, 18.0 percent of the city's medical force, up from 132, 14.9 percent in 1880.

This spate of five fictions within ten years suggests that the doctress, as she was then called, had not only attained public visibility, but had also captured the imagination. Access to medical education for women was a highly controversial issue after the middle of the century when they had begun to try to gain admission to regular medical schools. Women had always been informal healers within the kinship circle of family and neighbors; tendance of the sick had traditionally been an integral part of women's social function in their role as ministering angels in the house. Such self-help works as Dr. William Buchan's *Domestic Medicine; or a Treatise on the Prevention and Cure of Diseases by Regimen and Simple Remedies* (1772), *The Maternal Physician* (1818) by "An American Matron," and John G. Gunn's *Domestic Medicine* (1832) are all addressed to a female audience. In *A Country Doctor* Mrs. Martin Dyer is noted for her command of herbal remedies. Many nineteenth-century housekeeping manuals, such as the famous British work, Mrs. Beeton's *Book of Household Management* (1861) and the American Mary Mason's *The Young Housewife's Counsellor* (1871) offered not only recipes for invalid food but also extensive instructions on diagnosis and treatment of a large spectrum of disorders from fevers, animal and insect bites, and poisonings to such serious conditions as concussion, apoplexy, and epilepsy. Women were particularly prominent as midwives, as well as active in various sectarian health reform movements such as the then fashionable water-cures and the Physiological Societies, which taught the "laws of life" and hygiene to female audiences as an extension of domestic proficiency.

But this empirical exercise of paramedical skills was superseded in the course of the nineteenth century by the gradual rise and increasingly powerful organization of medicine as a profession, and, what is more, a distinctly *male* profession. The birth of scientific medicine together with the therapeutic revolution necessitated a more rigorous form of training than the instruction by apprenticeship that had been one of the usual ways to enter the profession in the earlier half of the century. So Nan in Jewett's novel undergoes formal training in medical school after an informal apprenticeship to Dr. Leslie. The growth of medical schools in the United States accelerated rapidly, rising in number from 52 in 1850 to 75 in 1870, 100 in 1880, 133 in 1890, and 160 by 1900. The duration and scope of the training was in the early 1870s extended through the addition of anatomy, physiology, chemistry, and pathological anatomy. The need to control the practice of medicine, and especially to protect the public from quacks, led to regulatory legislation, introduced successively into the American states as medical men converged in agreement that licensing was essential to ensure proper standards. This reform and institutionalization of medical education militated against women, who became casualties of medical professionalization. One woman, Elizabeth Blackwell, did achieve acceptance at the medical school in Geneva, New York in 1845 because faculty and students thought her application a joke and voted for it in jest; she graduated at the top of her class in 1849.

Women were excluded from medicine primarily for ideological reasons. The very idea of a woman being a *professional* doctor ran up against several deeply ingrained beliefs and prejudices of the period. Men and women were thought to have separate spheres of endeavor: the woman's in the domestic arena, and the man's in the public world. For a woman to work outside the home by choice was considered demeaning and "unladylike," although some intrepid women defied this prohibition in order to engage in such social causes as prison reform and the professionalization of nursing. Women were also regarded as physically too weak to stand the blood and agony of medicine, and as constitutionally "relative creatures," fitted to obey orders from men but not to take initiatives themselves. Finally, since medicine is essentially concerned with the body, the objections to women doctors also touched on the taboo on sexuality. However, this factor cut both ways; for the pioneering women aspirants to medicine argued for the need for female physicians on the grounds that many women were so reluctant to consult a male physician that they suffered unnecessarily and died prematurely. Women doctors aimed, in the words of Sophia Jex-Blake (1840–1912), one of the British leaders in the fight for women's admission to medical schools, to give "sisterly help and counsel"; they emphasized their intention of being of service to women and children.

Women were even deemed biologically unfit for education after puberty when all their energy should be directed to the development of what one physician described in 1895 as the "pelvic power" that would make them good mothers. That was the central argument, too, of Dr. Edward H. Clarke in his misleadingly titled treatise, *Sex in Education: A Fair Chance for Girls* (1873), in which he asserted that intellectual ac-

tivity during menstruation would surely lead to neuralgia, uterine disease, hysteria, and other derangements of the nervous system. The women,
for their part, were also ideologically motivated. Nan is "filled with energy
and a great desire for usefulness" (159), and excited by the "renown
some women physicians had and the avenues of usefulness which lay
open to her on every side" (193).

With the doors slammed in their faces, the women began to organize
their own medical colleges. The New England Female Medical College
opened in 1848, the Women's Medical College of Pennsylvania in Philadelphia in 1850, the New York Women's Medical College (homeopathic)
in 1863, the Homeopathic Medical College for Women in Cleveland in
1868, the Women's Medical College of the New York Infirmary for
Women and Children, and the Woman's Hospital Medical College in
Chicago in 1870, and the New York Free Medical College for Women
in 1871. None of these endeavors could have got off the ground without
the support and cooperation of some male physicians who were willing
to act as instructors until the women themselves had acquired sufficient
expertise and experience to teach their successors. Another serious problem was that of hands-on clinical instruction since women were denied
internships and residencies. So they founded dispensaries and hospitals
for women and children, of which the earliest were the New York Infirmary
for Women and Children, opened in 1857, and the New England Hospital for Women and Children in 1862. From these institutions the early
pioneer women doctors were graduated, including three black women:
Rebecca Lee in 1861, Rebecca Cole in 1867, and Sara McKinney Stewart
in 1870. Some of the more affluent and ambitious went on to further
training in those European universities that admitted women. Zurich,
open to women since 1864, was a popular destination; Nan is tempted
to go there, but decides to gain further experience at home first (252).
Paris, which admitted women in 1868, attracted women too, including
the British Elizabeth Garrett and the American Mary Putnam Jacobi,
who in 1870 and 1875, respectively, became the first two women to
attain the M.D. Back in the United States, well prepared to practice, the
doctresses faced more difficulties in obtaining membership in the state
medical associations. Such membership was not strictly a prerequisite for
practice; nevertheless, it had important practical implications as a symbol
of legitimate acceptance as well as for referrals, admission to hospital
staffs, in other words, for full integration into the profession. Curiously
evasive terms such as "inexpedient" and "inopportune" were advanced
for a while as grounds for rejection; the qualifications necessary for admission were declared to apply to males only. But in 1877 the state

societies of Kansas, Michigan, and Rhode Island did take women; others followed, with Massachussetts in 1884 among the last.

This then is the historical context for the fictional Nan's resolve to become a doctor. The novel illustrates throughout the opposition she encounters from various quarters. But she also has strong, sustained support from Dr. Leslie who is, despite his rather conservative views on the practice of medicine, very advanced in his social outlook. Nan's situation as an orphan proves an indirect advantage; like Elizabeth Stuart Phelps's Dr. Zay, parentless too, she is not subject to constant pressures from immediate family members with authority over her. Dr. Leslie is receptive to Nan's wishes (see "A Proper Vocation for Women"). Although he somewhat teasingly tells her that she "will be the successor to Mrs. Martin Dyer" (134), the herbalist, i.e., fulfilling the traditional womanly role, he quickly changes his tone to assure her that he will teach her all he can. Yet even he warns her that for a woman to study medicine is like "climbing a long hill" (134). Jewett gives no specific details about Nan's actual course of study in medical school, perhaps because she herself was unfamiliar with what that involved. Instead she focuses on the social aspects and philosophical arguments surrounding the question of women going into medicine.

Dr. Leslie's encouragement is the exception in Oldfields, where he and Nan live; as its name implies, it is a place where old attitudes prevail. When Dr. Leslie talks about Nan's future with his elderly neighbor, Mrs. Graham (chapter 10 of the novel: "Across the Street"), she is shocked at the degree of independence he is willing to grant his young ward, and expresses the conventional line in her response: "don't you think that a married life is the happiest?" (104). The same belief is expressed by Dr. Ferris, even though he has traveled far and wide. In his discussion with Dr. Leslie, he admonishes his old friend: "surely you don't mean to let her risk her happiness in following that career?" (see "Risking a Woman's Happiness"). He also warns Dr. Leslie not to "be disappointed when she's ten years older if she picks out a handsome young man and thinks there is nothing like housekeeping" (81).

Nan's severest test comes when she visits her aunt in Dunport. Miss Prince rejects in absolute horror the "silly notion" (described in the sixth selection) that Nan wants to practice medicine professionally as being wholly improper for a young woman of good family. Similar sentiments are expressed even more vehemently by Mrs. Fraley, a senior lady in Miss Prince's circle (see "Another Voice of Opposition"). Mrs. Fraley's maiden daughter, while secretly concurring with Nan, hardly dares to query her mother's opinions. In her timidity and submissiveness Eunice is a foil to the determined, bold Nan as well as a cautionary example of the emptiness of the life of a woman who remains unmarried and unoccupied.

During her stay at Dunport, Nan has another opportunity to demonstrate her medical skill and her growing knowledge when she goes to fetch water from a farm on a picnic and comes upon a farmer who has just suffered an acute shoulder injury (described in "Setting a Dislocated Shoulder Right"). She shows her presence of mind and her intrepidness in taking charge of the situation and repositioning the dislocated joint. Her rapid action and her success in this crisis serve to confirm her remarkable competence.

But at Dunport Nan also faces the temptation of giving up her goal and getting married when she meets the attractive young lawyer, George Gerry. After a sleepless night she decides that "I must do my part in my own way to make many homes happy instead of one" (242) even if this means "weariness and pain and reproach, and the loss of many things that other women held dearest and best" (229). Marriage, because it was considered the only suitable and desirable option for women in the nineteenth century, did indeed present a problem for the early doctresses. Some, notably the pioneer of medical education for women, Sophia Jex-Blake were adamantly opposed to women doctors marrying on the grounds that they could not simultaneously serve two masters, i.e., their family and their patients. On the other hand, a third to a fifth of women physicians did marry, often fellow physicians; some continued to practice, others chose not to. Is Nan making a wise decision in foregoing marriage? Will she regret her choice later? Given her temperament, how much choice does she really have? Would women at that time have been likely to empathize with her (as Eunice does) or to disapprove of her course of action?

Despite a certain streak of romance in the idealization of both Dr. Leslie and Nan, *A Country Doctor* gives a realistic picture of societal objections to women doctors in the later nineteenth century. It shows how social reality may hamper medical progress through ingrained prejudices. Jewett's novel uncovers those prejudices, and in so doing reveals their hollowness and irrationality. In order to make her plea for women doctors persuasive, Jewett has to endow Nan with exceptional gifts so that we may have no doubts that she will be an excellent practitioner.

Enter Dr. Leslie

Sarah Orne Jewett

The sick woman had refused to stay in the bedroom after she had come to her senses. She had insisted that she could not breathe, and that she was cold and must go back to the kitchen. Her mother and Mrs. Jake had wrapped her in blankets and drawn the high-backed wooden rocking chair close to the stove, and here she was just established when Mrs. Martin opened the outer door. Any one of less reliable nerves would have betrayed the shock which the sight of such desperate illness must have given. The pallor, the suffering, the desperate agony of the eyes, were far worse than the calmness of death, but Mrs. Martin spoke cheerfully, and even when her sister whispered that their patient had been attacked by a hemorrhage, she manifested no concern.

"How long has this be'n a-goin' on, Ad'line? Why didn't you come home before and get doctored up? You're all run down." Mrs. Thacher looked frightened when this questioning began, but turned her face toward her daughter, eager to hear the answer.

"I've been sick off and on all summer," said the young woman as if it were almost impossible to make the effort of speaking. "See if the baby's covered up warm, will you, Aunt 'Liza?"

"Yes, dear," said the kind-hearted woman, the tears starting to her eyes at the sound of the familiar affectionate fashion of speech which

From Sarah Orne Jewett, *A Country Doctor* (New York: New American Library, 1986), pp. 25–28.

Adeline had used in her childhood. "Don't you worry one mite; we're going to take care of you and the little gal too;" and then nobody spoke, while the only sound was the difficult breathing of the poor creature by the fire. She seemed like one dying, there was so little life left in her after her piteous homeward journey. The mother watched her eagerly with a mingled feeling of despair and comfort; it was terrible to have a child return in such sad plight, but it was a blessing to have her safe at home, and to be able to minister to her wants while life lasted.

They all listened eagerly for the sound of wheels, but it seemed a long time before Martin Dyer returned with the doctor. He had been met just as he was coming in from the other direction, and the two men had only paused while the tired horse was made comfortable, and a sleepy boy dispatched with the medicine for which he had long been waiting. The doctor's housekeeper had besought him to wait long enough to eat the supper which she had kept waiting, but he laughed at her and shook his head gravely, as if he already understood that there should be no delay. When he was fairly inside the Thacher kitchen, the benefaction of his presence was felt by every one. It was most touching to see the patient's face lose its worried look, and grow quiet and comfortable as if here were some one on whom she could entirely depend. The doctor's greeting was an every-day cheerful response to the women's welcome, and he stood for a minute warming his hands at the fire as if he had come upon a commonplace errand. There was something singularly self-reliant and composed about him; one felt that he was the wielder of great powers over the enemies, disease and pain, and that his brave hazel eyes showed a rare thoughtfulness and foresight. The rough driving coat which he had thrown off revealed a slender figure with the bowed shoulders of an untiring scholar. His head was finely set and scholarly, and there was that about him which gave certainty, not only of his sagacity and skill, but of his true manhood, his mastery of himself. Not only in this farm-house kitchen, but wherever one might place him, he instinctively took command, while from his great knowledge of human nature he could understand and help many of his patients whose aliments were not wholly physical. He seemed to read at a glance the shame and sorrow of the young woman who had fled to the home of her childhood, dying and worse than defeated, from the battle-field of life. And in this first moment he recognized with dismay the effects of that passion for strong drink which had been the curse of more than one of her ancestors. Even the pallor and the purifying influence of her mortal illness could not disguise these unmistakable signs.

"You can't do me any good, doctor," she whispered. "I shouldn't have let you come if it had been only that. I don't care how soon I am out of this world. But I want you should look after my little girl," and the poor soul watched the physician's face with keen anxiety as if she feared to see a shadow of unwillingness, but none came.

"I will do the best I can," and he still held her wrist, apparently thinking more of the fluttering pulse than of what poor Adeline was saying.

"That was what made me willing to come back," she continued, "you don't know how close I came to not doing it either. John will be good to her, but she will need somebody that knows the world better by and by. I wonder if you couldn't show me how to make out a paper giving you the right over her till she is of age? She must stay here with mother, long as she wants her. 'T is what I wish I had kept sense enough to do; life has not been all play to me;" and the tears began to roll quickly down the poor creature's thin cheeks. "The only thing I care about is leaving the baby well placed, and I want her to have a good chance to grow up a useful woman. And most of all to keep her out of *their* hands, his I mean her father's folks. I hate 'em, and he cared more for 'em than he did for *me,* long at the last of it. . . . I could tell you stories!"

"But not to-night, Addy," said the doctor gravely, as if he were speaking to a child. "We must put you to bed and to sleep, and you can talk about all these troublesome things in the morning. You shall see about the papers too, if you think best. Be a good girl now, and let your mother help you to bed." For the resolute spirit had summoned the few poor fragments of vitality that were left, and the sick woman was growing more and more excited. "You may have all the pillows you wish for, and sit up in bed if you like, but you mustn't stay here any longer," and he gathered her in his arms and quickly carried her to the next room. She made no resistance, and took the medicine which Mrs. Martin brought, without a word. There was a blazing fire now in the bedroom fire-place, and, as she lay still, her face took on a satisfied rested look. Her mother sat beside her, tearful, and yet contented and glad to have her near, and the others whispered together in the kitchen. It might have been the last night of a long illness instead of the sudden, startling entrance of sorrow in human shape. "No," said the doctor, "she cannot last much longer with such a cough as that, Mrs. Dyer. She has almost reached the end of it. I only hope that she will go quickly."

Practical Men versus Theorists

Sarah Orne Jewett

"If I settled myself into a respectable practice I should be obliged to march with the army of doctors who carry a great array of small weapons, and who find out what is the matter with their patients after all sorts of experiment and painstaking analysis, and comparing the results of their thermometers and microscopes with scientific books of reference. After I have done all that, you know, if I have had good luck I shall come to exactly what you can say before you have been with a sick man five minutes. You have the true gift for doctoring, you need no medical dictator, and whatever you study and whatever comes to you in the way of instruction simply ministers to your intuition. It grows to be a wonderful second-sight in such a man as you. I don't believe you investigate a case and treat it as a botanist does a strange flower, once a month. You know without telling yourself what the matter is, and what the special difference is, and the relative dangers of this case and one apparently just like it across the street, and you could do this before you were out of the hospitals. I remember you!" and after a few vigorous puffs of smoke he went on; "It is all very well for the rest of the men to be proud of their book learning, but they don't even try to follow nature, as Sydenham did, who followed no man. I believe such study takes one to more theory and scientific digest rather than to more skill. It is all very well to know

From Sarah Orne Jewett, *A Country Doctor* (New York: New American Library, 1986), pp. 81–83.

how to draw maps when one gets lost on a dark night, or even to begin with astronomical calculations and come down to a chemical analysis of the mud you stand in, but hang me if I wouldn't rather have the instinct of a dog who can go straight home across a bit of strange country. A man has no right to be a doctor if he doesn't simply make everything bend to his work of getting sick people well, and of trying to remedy the failures of strength that come from misuse or inheritance or ignorance. The anatomists and the pathologists have their place, but we must look to the living to learn the laws of life, not to the dead. A wreck shows you where the reef is, perhaps, but not how to manage a ship in the offing. The men who make it their business to write the books and the men who make it their business to follow them aren't the ones for successful practice."

Dr. Leslie smiled, and looked over his shoulder at his beloved library shelves, as if he wished to assure the useful volumes of his continued affection and respect, and said quietly, as if to beg the displeased surgeon's patience with his brethren: "They go on, poor fellows, studying the symptoms and never taking it in that the life power is at fault. I see more and more plainly that we ought to strengthen and balance the whole system, and aid nature to make the sick man well again. It is nature that does it after all, and diseases are oftener effects of illness than causes. But the young practitioners must follow the text-books a while until they have had enough experience to open their eyes to observe and have learned to think for themselves. I don't know which is worse; too much routine or no study at all. I was trying the other day to count up the different treatments of pneumonia that have been in fashion in our day; there must be seven or eight, and I am only afraid the next thing will be a sort of skepticism and contempt of remedies. Dr. Johnson said long ago that physicians were a class of men who put bodies of which they knew little into bodies of which they knew less, but certainly this isn't the fault of the medicines altogether; you and I know well enough they are often most stupidly used. If we blindly follow the medical dictators, as you call them, and spend our treatment on the effects instead of the causes, what success can we expect? We do want more suggestions from the men at work, but I suppose this is the same with every business. The practical medical men are the juries who settle all the theories of the hour, as they meet emergencies day after day."

Nan, the Young
"Assistant and Attendant"

Sara Orne Jewett

Nan, though eager to learn, and curious about many things in life and
nature, at first found her school lessons difficult, and sometimes came
appealingly to him [Dr. Leslie] for assistance, when circumstances had
made a temporary ending of her total indifference to getting the lessons
at all. For this and other reasons she sometimes sought the study, and
drew a small chair beside the doctor's large one before the blazing fire
of the black birch logs; and then Marilla [the housekeeper] in her turn
would venture upon the neutral ground between study and kitchen, and
smile with satisfaction at the cheerful companionship of the tired man
and the idle little girl who had already found her way to his lonely heart.
Nan had come to another home; there was no question about what
should be done with her and for her, but she was made free of the silent
old house, and went on growing taller, and growing dearer, and growing
happier day by day. Whatever the future might bring, she would be sure
to look back with love and longing to the first summer of her village life,
when, seeing that she looked pale and drooping, the doctor, to her
intense gratification, took her away from school. Presently, instead of
having a ride out into the country as an occasional favor, she might be
seen every day by the doctor's side, as if he could not make his morning

From Sarah Orne Jewett, *A Country Doctor* (New York: New American Library, 1986), pp.
65–67.

rounds without her; and in and out of the farmhouses she went, follow-ing him like a little dog, or, as Marilla scornfully expressed it, a briar at his heels; sitting soberly by when he dealt his medicines and gave advice, listening to his wise and merry talk with some, and his helpful advice and consolation to others of the country people. Many of these acquaintances treated Nan with great kindness; she half belonged to them, and was deeply interesting for the sake of her other ties of blood and bonds of fortune, while she took their courtesy with thankfulness, and their lack of notice with composure. If there were a shiny apple offered she was glad, but if not, she did not miss it, since her chief delight was in being the doctor's assistant and attendant, and her eyes were always watching for chances when she might be of use. And one day, coming out from a bedroom, the doctor discovered, to his amusement, that her quick and careful fingers had folded the papers of some powders which he had left unfolded on the table. As they drove home together in the bright noon sunshine, he said, as if the question were asked for the sake of joking a little, "What are you going to do when you grow up, Nan?" to which she answered gravely, as if it were the one great question of her life, "I should like best to be a doctor." Strangely enough there flitted through the doctor's mind a remembrance of the day when he had talked with Mrs. Meeker, and had looked up the lane to see the unlucky turkey whose leg had been put into splints. He had wished more than once that he had taken pains to see how the child had managed it; but old Mrs. Thacher had reported the case to have been at least partially successful.

Nan had stolen a look at her companion after the answer had been given, but had been pleased and comforted to find that he was not laughing at her, and at once began a lively picture of becoming famous in her chosen profession, and the valued partner of Dr. Leslie, whose skill everybody praised so heartily. He should not go out at night, and she would help him so much that he would wonder how he ever had been able to manage his wide-spread practice alone. It was a matter of no concern to her that Marilla had laughed when she had been told of Nan's intentions, and had spoken disrespectfully of women doctors; and the child's heart was full of pride and hope.

"A Proper Vocation for Women"?

Sarah Orne Jewett

The doctor was in such a hospitable frame of mind that nobody could have helped telling him anything, and happily he made an excellent introduction for Nan's secret by inquiring how she had got on with her studies, but she directed his attention to the wet plants in the bottom of the carriage, which were complimented before she said, a minute afterward, "Oh, I wonder if I shall make a mistake? I was afraid you would laugh at me, and think it was all nonsense."

"Dear me, no," replied the doctor. "You will be the successor of Mrs. Martin Dyer, and the admiration of the neighborhood;" but changing his tone quickly, he said: "I am going to teach you all I can, just as long as you have any wish to learn. It has not done you a bit of harm to know something about medicine, and I believe in your studying it more than you do yourself. I have always thought about it. But you are very young; there's plenty of time, and I don't mean to be hurried; you must remember that; though I see your fitness and peculiar adaptability a great deal better than you can these twenty years yet. You will be growing happier these next few years at any rate, however impossible life has seemed to you lately."

"I suppose there will be a great many obstacles," reflected Nan, with an absence of her usual spirit.

From Sarah Orne Jewett, *A Country Doctor* (New York: New American Library, 1986), pp. 133–135.

253

"Obstacles! Yes," answered Dr. Leslie vigorously. "Of course there will be; it is climbing a long hill to try to study medicine or to study anything else. And if you are going to fear obstacles you will have a poor chance at success. There are just as many reasons as you will stop to count up why you should not do your plain duty, but if you are going to make anything of yourself you must go straight ahead, taking it for granted that there will be opposition enough, but doing what is right all the same. I suppose I have repeated to you fifty times what old Friend Meadows told me years ago; he was a great success at money-making, and once I asked him to give me some advice about a piece of property. 'Friend Leslie,' says he, 'thy own opinion is the best for thee; if thee asks ten people what to do, they will tell thee ten things, and then thee doesn't know as much as when thee set out,'" and Dr. Leslie, growing very much in earnest, reached forward for the whip. "I want you to be a good woman, and I want you to be all the use you can," he said. "It seems to me like stealing, for men and women to live in the world and do nothing to make it better. You have thought a great deal about this, and so have I, and now we will do the best we can at making a good doctor of you. I don't care whether people think it is a proper vocation for women or not. It seems to me that it is more than proper for you, and God has given you a fitness for it which it is a shame to waste. And if you ever hesitate and regret what you have said, you won't have done yourself any harm by learning how to take care of your own health and other people's."

"But I shall never regret it," said Nan stoutly. "I don't believe I should ever be fit for anything else, and you know as well as I that I must have something to do. I used to wish over and over again that I was a boy, when I was a little thing down at the farm, and the only reason I had in the world was that I could be a doctor, like you."

"Better than that, I hope," said Dr. Leslie. "But you mustn't think it will be a short piece of work; it will take more patience than you are ready to give just now, and we will go on quietly and let it grow by the way, like your waterweed here."

Risking a Woman's Happiness?

Sarah Orne Jewett

"How about the little girl herself?" asked the guest presently; "she seems well combined, and likely, as they used to say when I was a boy."

Dr. Leslie resumed the subject willingly: "So far as I can see, she has the good qualities of all her ancestors without the bad ones. Her mother's mother was an old fashioned country woman of the best stock. Of course she resented what she believed to be her daughter's wrongs, and refused to have anything to do with her son-in-law's family, and kept the child as carefully as possible from any knowledge of them. Little Nan was not strong at first, but I insisted that she should be allowed to run free out of doors. It seems to me that up to seven or eight years of age children are simply bundles of inheritances, and I can see the traits of one ancestor after another; but a little later than the usual time she began to assert her own individuality, and has grown capitally well in mind and body ever since. There is an amusing trace of the provincial self-reliance and self-respect and farmer-like dignity, added to a quick instinct, and tact and ready courtesy, which must have come from the other side of her ancestry. She is more a child of the soil than any country child I know, and yet she would not put a city household to shame. She has seen nothing of the world of course, but you can see she isn't like the usual village school-girl. There is one thing quite remarkable. I believe she has

From Sarah Orne Jewett, *A Country Doctor* (New York: New American Library, 1986), pp. 77–78, 79–81.

255

grown up as naturally as a plant grows, not having been clipped back or forced in any unnatural direction. If ever a human being were untrammeled and left alone to see what will come of it, it is this child. And I will own I am very much interested to see what will appear later."

The navy surgeon's eyes twinkled at this enthusiasm, but he asked soberly what seemed to be our heroine's bent, so far as could be discovered, and laughed outright when he was gravely told that it was a medical bent; a surprising understanding of things pertaining to that most delightful profession.

"But you surely don't mean to let her risk her happiness in following that career?" Dr. Ferris inquired with feigned anxiety for his answer. "You surely aren't going to sacrifice that innocent creature to a theory! I know it's a theory; last time I was here, you could think of nothing but hypnotism or else the action of belladonna in congestion and inflammation of the brain;" and he left his very comfortable chair suddenly, with a burst of laughter, and began to walk up and down the room. "She has no relatives to protect her, and I consider it a shocking case of a guardian's inhumanity. Grown up naturally indeed! I don't doubt that you supplied her with Bells 'Anatomy' for a picture-book and made her say over the names of the eight little bones of her wrist, instead of 'This little pig went to market.'"

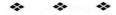

"Are you going to fit your ward for general practice or for a specialty?"

"I don't know; that'll be for the young person herself to decide," said Dr. Leslie good-humoredly. "But she's showing a real talent for medical matters. It is quite unconscious for the most part, but I find that she understands a good deal already, and she sat here all the afternoon last week with one of my old medical dictionaries. I couldn't help looking over her shoulder as I went by, and she was reading about fevers, if you please, as if it were a story-book. I didn't think it was worth while to tell her we understood things better nowadays, and didn't think it best to bleed as much as old Dr. Rush recommended."

"You're like a hen with one chicken, Leslie," said the friend, still pacing to and fro. "But seriously, I like your notion of her having come to this of her own accord. Most of us are grown in the shapes that society and family preference and prejudice fasten us into, and don't find out until we are well toward middle life that we should have done a great deal better at something else. Our vocations are likely enough to be badly chosen, since few persons are fit to choose them for us, and we are at the most unreasonable stage of life when we choose them for ourselves. And what the Lord made some people for, nobody ever can understand; some of us are for use and more are for waste, like the flowers. I am in such a hurry to know what the next world is like that I can hardly wait to get to it. Good heavens! we live here in our familiar fashion, going at a jog-trot pace round our little circles, with only a friend or two to speak with who understand us, and a pipe and a jack-knife and a few books and some old clothes, and please ourselves by thinking we know the universe! Not a soul of us can tell what it is that sends word to our little fingers to move themselves back and forward."

"We're sure of two things at any rate," said Dr. Leslie, "love to God and love to man. And though I have lived here all my days, I have learned some truths just as well as if I had gone about with you, or even been to the next world and come back. I have seen too many lives go to pieces, and too many dissatisfied faces, and I have heard too many sorrowful confessions from these country death-beds I have watched beside, one after another, for twenty or thirty years. And if I can help one good child to work with nature and not against it, and to follow the lines marked out for her, and she turns out useful and intelligent, and keeps off the rocks of mistaking her duty, I shall be more than glad. I don't care whether it's a man's work or a woman's work; if it is hers I'm going to help her the very best way I can. I don't talk to her of course; she's much too young; but I watch her and mean to put the things in her way that she seems to reach out for and try to find. She is going to be very practical, for her hands can almost always work out her ideas already. I like to see her take hold of things, and I like to see her walk and the way she lifts her feet and puts them down again. I must say, Ferris, there is a great satisfaction in finding a human being once in a while that has some use of itself."

"You're right!" said Dr. Ferris—"but don't be disappointed when she's ten years older if she picks out a handsome young man and thinks there is nothing like housekeeping."

"A Silly Notion"?

Sarah Orne Jewett

Nan stopped her hand as it reached for the cup which Miss Prince had just filled. "School; yes," she answered, somewhat bewildered; "but you know I am studying medicine." This most important of all facts had been so present to her own mind, even in the excitement and novelty of her new surroundings, that she could not understand that her aunt was still entirely ignorant of the great purpose of her life.

"What do you mean?" demanded Miss Prince, coldly, and quickly explained to their somewhat amused and astonished companion, "My niece has been the ward of a distinguished physician, and it is quite natural she should have become interested in his pursuits."

"But I am really studying medicine; it is to be my profession," persisted Nan fearlessly, though she was sorry that she had spoiled the harmony of the little company. "And my whole heart is in it, Aunt Nancy."

"Nonsense, my dear," returned Miss Prince, who had recovered her self-possession partially. "Your father gave promise of attaining great eminence in a profession that was very proper for him, but I thought better of Dr. Leslie than this. I cannot understand his indulgence of such a silly notion."

From Sarah Orne Jewett, *A Country Doctor* (New York: New American Library, 1986), pp. 185–186.

George Gerry felt very uncomfortable. He had been a good deal shocked, but he had a strong impulse to rush into the field as Nan's champion, though it were quite against his conscience. She had been too long in a humdrum country-town with no companion but an elderly medical man. And after a little pause he made a trifling joke about their making the best of the holiday, and the talk was changed to other subjects. The tide was strong against our heroine, but she had been assailed before, and had no idea of sorrowing yet over a lost cause. And for once Miss Prince was in a hurry for Mr. Gerry to go away.

Another Voice of Opposition

Sarah Orne Jewett

"In my time," Mrs. Fraley continued, "it was thought proper for young women to show an interest in household affairs. When I was married it was not asked whether I was acquainted with dissecting-rooms."

"But I don't think there is any need of that," replied Nan. "I think such things are the duty of professional men and women only. I am very far from believing that every girl ought to be a surgeon any more than that she ought to be an astronomer. And as for the younger people's being less strong than the old, I am afraid it is their own fault, since we understand the laws of health better than we used. 'Who breaks, pays,' you know."

It was evidently not expected that the young guest should venture to discuss the question, but rather have accepted her rebuke meekly, and acknowledged herself in the wrong. But she had the courage of her opinions, and the eagerness of youth, and could hardly bear to be so easily defeated. So when Mrs. Fraley, mistaking the moment's silence for a final triumph, said again, that a woman's place was at home, and that a strong-minded woman was out of place, and unwelcome everywhere, the girl's cheeks flushed suddenly.

"I think it is a pity that we have fallen into a habit of using strong-mindedness as a term of rebuke," she said. "I am willing to acknowledge

From Sarah Orne Jewett, *A Country Doctor* (New York: New American Library, 1986), pp. 207–211.

that people who are eager for reforms are apt to develop unpleasant traits, but it is only because they have to fight against opposition and ignorance. When they are dead and the world is reaping the reward of their bravery and constancy, it no longer laughs, but makes statues of them, and praises them, and thanks them in every way it can. I think we ought to judge each other by the highest standards, Mrs. Fraley, and by whether we are doing good work."

"My day is past," said the hostess. "I do not belong to the present, and I suppose my judgment is worth nothing to you;" and Nan looked up quickly and affectionately.

"I should like to have all my friends believe that I am doing right," she said. "I do feel very certain that we must educate people properly if we want them to be worth anything. It is no use to treat all the boys and girls as if nature had meant them for the same business and scholarship, and try to put them through the same drill, for that is sure to mislead and confuse all those who are not perfectly sure of what they want. There are plenty of people dragging themselves miserably through the world, because they are clogged and fettered with work for which they have no fitness. I know I haven't had the experience that you have, Mrs. Fraley, but I can't help believing that nothing is better than to find one's work early and hold fast to it, and put all one's heart into it."

"I have done my best to serve God in the station to which it has pleased Him to call me," said Mrs. Fraley, stiffly. "I believe that a young man's position is very different from a girl's. To be sure, I can give my opinion that everything went better when the master workmen took apprentices to their trades, and there wasn't so much schooling. But I warn you, my dear, that your notion about studying to be a doctor has shocked me very much indeed. I could not believe my ears,—a refined girl who bears an honorable and respected name to think of being a woman doctor! If you were five years older you would never have dreamed of such a thing. It lowers the pride of all who have any affection for you. If it were not that your early life had been somewhat peculiar and most unfortunate, I should blame you more; as it is, I can but wonder at the lack of judgment in others. I shall look forward in spite of it all to seeing you happily married." To which Miss Prince assented with several decided nods.

"This is why I made up my mind to be a physician," said the culprit; and though she had been looking down and growing more uncomfortable every moment, she suddenly gave her head a quick upward movement and looked at Mrs. Fraley frankly, with a beautiful light in her clear eyes. "I believe that God has given me a fitness for it, and that I never could do anything else half so well. Nobody persuaded me into following such a plan; I simply grew toward it. And I have everything to learn, and a great many faults to overcome, but I am trying to get on as fast as may be. I can't be too glad that I have spent my childhood in a way that has helped me to use my gift instead of hindering it. But everything helps a young man to follow his bent; he has an honored place in society, and just because he is a student of one of the learned professions, he ranks above the men who follow other pursuits. I don't see why it should be a shame and dishonor to a girl who is trying to do the same thing and to be of equal use in the world. God would not give us the same talents if what were right for men were wrong for women."

"My dear, it is quite unnatural you see," said the antagonist, impatiently. "Here you are less than twenty-five years old, and I shall hear of your being married next thing,—at least I hope I shall,—-and you will laugh at all this nonsense. A woman's place is at home. Of course I know that there have been some women physicians who have attained eminence, and some artists, and all that. But I would rather see a daughter of mine take a more retired place. The best service to the public can be done by keeping one's own house in order and one's husband comfortable, and by attending to those social responsibilities which come in our way. The mothers of the nation have rights enough and duties enough already, and need not look farther than their own firesides, or wish for the plaudits of an ignorant public."

"But if I do not wish to be married, and do not think it right that I should be," said poor Nan at last. "If I have good reasons against all that, would you have me bury the talent God has given me, and choke down the wish that makes itself a prayer every morning that I may do this work lovingly and well? It is the best way I can see of making myself useful in the world. People must have good health or they will fail of reaching what success and happiness are possible for them; and so many persons might be better and stronger than they are now, which would make their lives very different. I do think if I can help my neighbors in this way it will be a great kindness. I won't attempt to say that the study of medicine is a proper vocation for women, only that I believe more and more every year that it is the proper study for me. It certainly cannot be the proper vocation of all women to bring up children, so many of them are dead failures at it; and I don't see why all girls should be thought failures who do not marry. I don't believe that half those who do marry have any real right to it, at least until people use common sense as much in that most important decision as in lesser ones. Of course we can't expect to bring about an ideal state of society all at once; but just because we don't really believe in having the best possible conditions, we make no effort at all toward even better ones. People ought to work with the great laws of nature and not against them."

"You don't know anything about it," said Mrs. Fraley, who hardly knew what to think of this ready opposition. "You don't know what you are talking about, Anna. You have neither age nor experience, and it is easy to see you have been associating with very foolish people. I am the last person to say that every marriage is a lucky one; but if you were my daughter I should never consent to your injuring your chances for happiness in this way."

Nan could not help stealing a glance at poor Miss Eunice, behind her fragile battlement of the tea-set, and was deeply touched at the glance of sympathy which dimly flickered in the lonely eyes. "I do think, mother, that Anna is right about single women's having some occupation," was timidly suggested. "Of course, I mean those who have no special home duties."

Setting a Dislocated Shoulder

Sarah Orne Jewett

There did not seem to be anybody in the kitchen into which they could look through the open doorway, though they could hear steps and voices from some part of the house beyond it; and it was not until they had knocked again loudly that a woman came to answer them, looking worried and pale.

"I never was so glad to see folks, though I don't know who you be," she said hurriedly. "I believe I shall have to ask you to go for help. My man's got hurt; he managed to get home, but he's broke his shoulder, or any ways 't is out o' place. He was to the pasture, and we've got some young cattle, and somehow or 'nother one he'd caught and was meaning to lead home give a jump, and John lost his balance; he says he can't see how 't should 'a' happened, but over he went and got jammed against a rock before he could let go o' the rope he'd put round the critter's neck. He's in dreadful pain so 't I couldn't leave him, and there's nobody but me an' the baby. You'll have to go to the next house and ask them to send; Doctor Bent's always attended of us."

"Let me see him," said Nan with decision. "Wait a minute, Mr. Gerry, or perhaps you had better come in too," and she led the way, while the surprised young man and the mistress of the house followed

---

From Sarah Orne Jewett, *A Country Doctor* (New York: New American Library, 1986), pp. 197–199.

her. The patient was a strong young fellow, who sat on the edge of the bed in the little kitchen bedroom, pale as ashes, and holding one elbow with a look of complete misery, though he stopped his groans as the strangers came in.

"Lord bless you, young man! don't wait here," he said; "tell the doctor it may only be out o' place, but I feel as if 't was broke."

But Nan had taken a pair of scissors from the high mantelpiece and was making a cut in the coarse, white shirt, which was already torn and stained by its contact with the ground, and with quick fingers and a look of deep interest made herself sure what had happened, when she stood still for a minute and seemed a little anxious, and all at once entirely determined. "Just lie down on the floor a minute," she said, and the patient with some exclamations, but no objections, obeyed.

Nan pushed the spectators into the doorway of the kitchen, and quickly stooped and unbuttoned her right boot, and then planted her foot on the damaged shoulder and caught up the hand and gave a quick pull, the secret of which nobody understood; but there was an unpleasant cluck as the bone went back into its socket, and a yell from the sufferer, who scrambled to his feet.

"I'll be hanged if she ain't set it," he said, looking quite weak and very much astonished. "You're the smartest young woman I ever see. I shall have to lay down just to pull my wits together. Marthy, a drink of water," and by the time this was brought the excitement seemed to be at an end, though the patient was a little faint, and his wife looked at Nan admiringly. Nan herself was fastening her boot again with unwonted composure. George Gerry had not a word to say, and listened to a simple direction of Nan's as if it were meant for him, and acceded to her remark that she was glad for the shoulder's sake that it did not have to wait and grow worse and worse all the while the doctor was being brought from town. And after a few minutes when the volley of thanks and compliments could be politely cut short, the two members of the picnic party set forth with their pail of water to join their companions.

"Will you be so good as to tell me how you knew enough to do that?" asked Mr. Gerry humbly, and looking at his companion with admiration. "I should not have had the least idea."

"I was very glad it turned out so well," said Nan simply. "It was a great pleasure to be of use, they were so frightened, poor things. We won't say anything about it, will we?"

But the young man did not like to think yet of the noise the returning bone had made. He was stouthearted enough usually; as brave a fellow as one could wish to see; but he felt weak and womanish, and somehow wished it had been he who could play the doctor. Nan hurried back bareheaded to the oak grove as if nothing had happened, though, if possible, she looked gayer and brighter than ever. And when the waiting party scolded a little at their slow pace, Miss Prince was much amused and made two or three laughing apologies for their laziness, and even ventured to give the information that they had made a pleasant call at the farm-house.

13

A Shocking Discovery!

An Introduction to Arthur Conan Doyle's "The Doctors of Hoyland"

Arthur Conan Doyle (1859–1930) is renowned as the creator of Sherlock Holmes; less well known is the fact that he was a qualified doctor. Lacking capital, he had a hard struggle to get established in the profession; in *The Stark Munro Letters* (1895) he describes in an amusing way the difficulties of a young, impecunious physician, like himself, as he goes through a series of positions as an assistant in a large practice, as a resident caretaker to a lord's insane son, as a ship's surgeon, etc. Near the beginning of "The Doctors of Hoyland" mention is made of three successive doctors who had tried to set up practice in the town and had given up, thus underscoring the problems of getting established. Dr. Ripley, as we hear in the story's opening sentence, has the immense advantage of having followed his father into the practice. In the long hours of waiting for patients, Conan Doyle began to write so as to supplement his income. With the publication of the first of the Sherlock Holmes stories, *A Study in Scarlet* (1887), he found that he could make a more lucrative and easier living with the pen than with the stethoscope.

"The Doctors of Hoyland" is one of fifteen stories with medical themes collected in *Round the Red Lamp* (1894). A red lamp, hung outside a house, was used in late-nineteenth-century Britain to signal the presence of a doctor and to guide patients after dark and on foggy days. All the stories are short; most of them deal with encounters between doctor and patient in a serious tone. Generally also they portray physicians in a favorable light, showing the alleviation of pain and the comfort they are able to bring, although in "The Third Generation" the lure of his research momentarily distracts the doctor from attention to a patient when he comes to see him as an example of an interesting, unusual syndrome.

Conan Doyle is fully aware of the authority conferred by the new scientific instruments; in "A Question of Diplomacy," "a doctor with his stethoscope and thermometer" is described as "a thing apart" with whom no one can argue (182). On the other hand, the practitioner in "Behind the Times" scorns even the stethoscope as "a new-fangled French toy" (4), yet "his patients do very well. He has the healing touch" so that "his mere presence leaves the patient with more hopefulness and vitality" (6). Conan Doyle shows here the older physician's skepticism about new methods and instruments as well as patients' preference for simpler, tried remedies, backed by the doctor's charismatic personality. The story ends in a comical vein as the two young doctors, who had discoursed learnedly about mitral murmurs and bronchitic rales (sounds heard with a stethoscope), themselves call in the empathetic old practitioner when they are struck by a bad attack of influenza. On the other hand, "The Doctors of Hoyland" endorses the efficacy of innovative techniques and the value of research in the cures that Dr. Smith achieves.

"The Doctors of Hoyland" stands out from the majority of the stories in *Round the Red Lamp* for its satirical edge and its ironical sting-in-the-tail. It is the most jovial of a cluster of fictions that appeared in England between 1877 and the early 1890s about the controversial figure of the woman doctor, corresponding to the similar cluster in the United States: Charles Reade, *A Woman-Hater* (1877), G. G. Alexander, *Dr. Victoria: A Picture from the Period* (1881), the anonymously published *Dr. Edith Romney* (1883), and *Mona Maclean: Medical Student* (1891) by "Graham Travers," the pseudonym of Margaret Georgiana Todd, who was Jex-Blake's biographer.

In Great Britain the struggle by women to gain access to medical schools and to become professional physicians took place along lines parallel to those in the United Sates, running up against the same type of objections. However, the actual sequence of events was somewhat different. A major landmark in the history of British medicine is the Medical Registration Act (1858) and the subsequent establishment of the Medical Register (1859), which forged the profession's identity by welding practitioners into a body with rights and responsibilities. Though not directed specifically against women, the new law had the effect of debarring them because it named the possession of a degree from a British university as the required qualification. Since women were not admitted to universities, the Act represented a *de facto* block on the possibility of medical education for women. Jex-Blake, writing in 1886 in "Medicine as a Profession for Women" in *Medical Women*, argued persuasively that the innovation lay in the exclusion of women from the sphere of healing in which they had previously participated. The 1858 Act, she maintains,

> was wrested from its original purpose, and made an almost in-
> surmountable barrier to the admission of women to the autho-
> rized practice of medicine; and this because the Act made it
> obligatory on all candidates to comply with certain conditions,
> and yet left it in the power of the Medical Schools, collectively,
> arbitrarily to preclude women from such compliance. (65)

Only one woman was listed in the 1859 Register: Elizabeth Blackwell (1821–1910), who was included under the provision admitting anyone with a foreign degree already practicing in England in 1858. Blackwell had in 1849 graduated top of her class at the Medical School in Geneva, New York. Elizabeth Garrett Anderson (1836–1917) also succeeded in being listed on the Medical Register in 1865 by making use of a loop-hole in the system to obtain a license granted under the 1815 Apothecaries' Act. This loophole was then promptly closed by a ban forbidding students to receive any part of their education privately. Jex-Blake's own attempts to get into Harvard in 1867, together with the American Susan Dimock, who later became an eminent surgeon, met with resounding opposition despite both applicants' good preparation, extensive lobby-ing, and significant support from some male faculty members. Resilient and persistent, Jex-Blake re-applied to Harvard in 1868, and tried Lon-don as well before turning her attention to Edinburgh on account of its reputation for enlightened views regarding education. The tumultuous struggle for admission and full acceptance that took place in Edinburgh between 1869 and 1873 is vividly chronicled, day by day and blow by blow, by Jex-Blake in "The Medical Education of Women," and told in fictionalized form in Reade's *A Woman-Hater*, whose heroine is por-trayed as one of the seven women who tried to storm their way into the Edinburgh medical school. But this initiative, too, ended in failure with scandals, lawsuits, and the women's retreat by March 1874.

The London School of Medicine for Women was finally established in 1874, and in 1876 a law was enacted permitting women to practice.

Between 1877 and 1885 forty-eight women were entered onto the British Medical Register, and by 1886 women's dispensaries (outpatient clinics) and hospitals had been established in many major British cities.

This is the historical context for Conan Doyle's story. From the mention of pamphlets published in 1890 and 1891, we can assume that the time of the action is shortly prior to its appearance in 1894. By then women were just beginning to make their presence felt in medicine, although they were still a relative rarity. Seeing that his new competitor in Hoyland had studied with distinction at the foremost medical schools in Edinburgh, Paris, Berlin, and Vienna, and had been awarded a gold medal and a scholarship for research, Dr. Ripley naturally assumes that the newcomer must be a *man*. His mistake is facilitated by Dr. Smith's unusual first name, "Verrinder," which is free of gender associations. Conan Doyle cleverly makes the whole story hinge on the misapprehension fostered by this name. Dr. Smith's status as an upstart intruder is underscored by Dr. Ripley's own hereditary lineage as his father's successor in the Hoyland practice.

While waiting for Dr. Smith at his initial visit, Dr. Ripley notices "elaborate instruments" and "a book-case full of ponderous volumes in French and German." These details indicate Dr. Smith's scientific interests which match Dr. Ripley's own (he dissects sheep's eyes), and raise his hopes of a congenial partner for "long evenings of high scientific talk." These hopes are shattered by his deeply shocking discovery that Dr. Smith is a *woman*. Dr. Ripley completely loses his composure and his temper; afterwards he realizes that "he had come very badly out of it" on account both of his rude behavior and her superior knowledge of the latest research findings. At this first encounter already Dr. Smith gains the upper hand through her unruffled politeness (befitting a lady), and her impressive command of medicine. Her scholarly acumen places her squarely on the side of science in the debate about the style of medicine that women should practice. Elizabeth Blackwell believed that it should differ from male medicine in being gentler ("maternal" was her term) whereas the distinguished American physician, Mary Putnam Jacobi, strongly favored the scientific model.

But Dr. Smith is not merely a brilliant theoretical researcher. She proves her practical competence in attending expertly on Dr. Ripley's broken leg. With a "dexterity" described as "masterly," she performs on a child's club foot the very surgery that ended so disastrously in *Madame Bovary*. Nevertheless, her rapid conquest of the country folk as she drains patients away from Dr. Ripley is hard to believe. Her immediate, startling success contrasts with the failure of her three predecessors in Hoyland,

and is the more astonishing in light of the prejudices against women doctors. Her boldness is further emphasized when she treats a male patient, admittedly in an emergency, thereby transgressing the convention that female physicians attended to women and children.

With her "plain, palish face," her slight stature, and her *pince-nez* (spectacles), Dr. Smith does not at first glance appear to be an attractive woman except for her remarkably shrewd, humorous, blue-green eyes. Set in his rejection of women doctors without ever having actually met one, Dr. Ripley dismisses (and insults) her as typical of the "masculine ladies" in medicine. Here he voices the notion current at the time that study would rob a young woman of her charm as well as of her health. He elevates the issue from a practical to an ethical, even metaphysical level by feeling "as if a blasphemy had been committed," yet he cannot recall any Biblical injunction against women doctors. This reference to Biblical imperatives shows just how very seriously the presence of female physicians was taken, and how radically threatening they seemed to be to the established moral as well as social order. When Dr. Ripley's brother from London expresses the same derogatory opinions, the pervasiveness of these men's views is further confirmed.

By the time of his brother's visit, Dr. Ripley has already begun to modify his attitude. He is struck by Dr. Smith's medical competence in managing a crisis; she does not lose her head in an emergency, as his brother thinks women doctors are likely to do. Even earlier he had noticed her "bright, mobile face," "humorous eyes," and "strong, well-turned chin." He comes to look forward to her professional visits during the weeks that his leg is mending, and finally realizes that he has fallen for her charms.

So in "The Doctors of Hoyland" a neat, but profound reversal takes place in Dr. Ripley's stance toward Dr. Smith and the whole question of women doctors. We as readers are made to share his conversion because the story is narrated through *his* eyes. We do not hear what Dr. Smith thinks of Dr. Ripley so that the ending is a second shocking discovery, a symmetrical counterpart to the earlier one. On the surface a wrily comic tale, "The Doctors of Hoyland" is a masterpiece of the genre of the short story. its brevity, use of dramatic dialogue, and skillful handling of narrative perspective create the fast movement and repeated surprise that hold readers' attention. Yet it also raises some thorny questions: are the reactions of Dr. Ripley and his brother too extreme? Is Dr. Smith too perfect, too much an idealized, exaggerated figure (like Dr. Leslie and Nan in Jewett's *A Country Doctor* [chapter 12])? Is the story in a way sad as well as humorous? Would a happy ending in marriage and professional partnership be seen as an anticlimax, or would readers, then and now, prefer it? Is "The Doctors of Hoyland" potentially a fairytale, inverted because it does not work out? Does this undermine its interest as a reflection of a social reality?

"The Doctors of Hoyland"

Arthur Conan Doyle

Dr. James Ripley was always looked upon as an exceedingly lucky dog by all who knew him. His father has preceded him in a practice in the village of Hoyland, in the north of Hampshire, and all was ready for him on the very first day that the law allowed him to put his name at the foot of a prescription. In a few years the old gentleman retired, and settled on the South Coast, leaving his son in undisputed possession of the whole country side. Save for Dr. Horton, near Basingstoke, the young surgeon had a clear run of six miles in every direction, and took his fifteen hundred pounds a year, though, as is usual in country practices, the stable swallowed up most of what the consulting-room earned.

Dr. James Ripley was two-and-thirty years of age, reserved, learned, unmarried, with set, rather stern features, and a thinning of the dark hair upon the top of his head, which was worth quite a hundred a year to him. He was particularly happy in his management of ladies. He had caught the tone of bland sternness and decisive suavity which dominates without offending. Ladies, however, were not equally happy in their management of him. Professionally, he was always at their service. Socially, he was a drop of quicksilver. In vain the country mammas spread out their simple lures in front or him. Dances and picnics were not to his taste, and he preferred during his scanty leisure to shut himself up in

From Arthur Conan Doyle, *Round the Red Lamp* (London: Methuen, 1894), pp. 295–315.

his study, and to bury himself in Virchow's Archives and the professional journals.

Study was a passion with him, and he would have none of the rust which often gathers round a country practitioner. It was his ambition to keep his knowledge as fresh and bright as at the moment when he had stepped out of the examination hall. He prided himself on being able at a moment's notice to rattle off the seven ramifications of some obscure artery, or to give the exact percentage of any physiological compound. After a long day's work he would sit up half the night performing iridectomies and extractions upon the sheep's eyes sent in by the village butcher, to the horror of his housekeeper, who had to remove the *debris* next morning. His love for his work was the one fanaticism which found a place in his dry, precise nature.

It was the more to his credit that he should keep up to date in his knowledge, since he had no competition to force him to exertion. In the seven years during which he had practised in Hoyland three rivals had pitted themselves against him, two in the village itself and one in the neighbouring hamlet of Lower Hoyland. Of these one had sickened and wasted, being, as it was said, himself the only patient whom he had treated during his eighteen months of ruralising. A second had bought a fourth share of a Basingstoke practice, and had departed honourably, while a third had vanished one September night, leaving a gutted house and an unpaid drug bill behind him. Since then the district had become a monopoly, and no one had dared to measure himself against the established fame of the Hoyland doctor.

It was, then, with a feeling of some surprise and considerable curiosity that on driving through Lower Hoyland one morning he perceived that the new house at the end of the village was occupied, and that a virgin brass plate glistened upon the swinging gate which faced the high road. He pulled up his fifty guinea chestnut mare and took a good look at it. "Verrinder Smith, M.D.," was printed across it in very neat, small lettering. The last man had had letters half a foot long, with a lamp like a fire-station. Dr. James Ripley noted the difference, and deduced from it that the newcomer might possibly prove a more formidable opponent. He was convinced of it that evening when he came to consult the current medical directory. By it he learned that Dr. Verrinder Smith was the holder of superb degrees, that he had studied with distinction at Edinburgh, Paris, Berlin, and Vienna. and finally that he had been awarded a gold medal and the Lee Hopkins scholarship for original research, in recognition of an exhaustive inquiry into the functions of the anterior spinal nerve roots. Dr. Ripley passed his fingers through his thin hair in bewilderment as he read his rival's record. What on earth would so brilliant a man mean by putting up his plate in a little Hampshire hamlet.

But Dr. Ripley furnished himself with an explanation to the riddle. No doubt Dr. Verrinder Smith had simply come down there in order to pursue some scientific research in peace and quiet. The plate was up as an address rather than as an invitation to patients. Of course, that must be the true explanation. In that case the presence of this brilliant neighbour would be a splendid thing for his own studies. He had often longed for some kindred mind, some steel on which he might strike his flint. Chance had brought it to him, and he rejoiced exceedingly.

And this joy it was which led him to take a step which was quite at variance with his usual habits. It is the custom for a new-comer among medical men to call first upon the older, and the etiquette upon the subject is strict. Dr. Ripley was pedantically exact on such points, and yet he deliberately drove over next day and called upon Dr. Verrinder Smith. Such a waiving of ceremony was, he felt, a gracious act upon his part, and a fit prelude to the intimate relations which he hoped to establish with his neighbour.

The house was neat and well appointed, and Dr. Ripley was shown by a smart maid into a dapper little consulting room. As he passed in he noticed two or three parasols and a lady's sun bonnet hanging in the hall. It was a pity that his colleague should be a married man. It would put them upon a different footing, and interfere with those long evenings of high scientific talk which he had pictured to himself. On the other hand, there was much in the consulting room to please him. Elaborate instruments, seen more often in hospitals than in the houses of private practitioners, were scattered about. A sphygmograph stood upon the table and a gasometer-like engine, which was new to Dr. Ripley, in the corner. A book-case full of ponderous volumes in French and German, paper-covered for the most part, and varying in tint from the shell to the yoke of a duck's egg, caught his wandering eyes, and he was deeply absorbed in their titles when the door opened suddenly behind him. Turning round, he found himself facing a little woman, whose plain, palish face was remarkable only for a pair of shrewd, humorous eyes of a blue which had two shades too much green in it. She held a *pince-nez* in her left hand, and the doctor's card in her right.

"How do you do, Dr. Ripley?" said she.

"How do you do, madam?" returned the visitor. "Your husband is perhaps out?"

"I am not married," said she simply.

"Oh, I beg your pardon! I meant the doctor—Dr. Verrinder Smith."

"I am Dr. Verrinder Smith."

Dr. Ripley was so surprised that he dropped his hat and forgot to pick it up again.

"What!" he gasped, "the Lee Hopkins prizeman! You!"

He had never seen a woman doctor before, and his whole conservative soul rose up in revolt at the idea. He could not recall any Biblical injunction that the man should remain ever the doctor and the woman the nurse, and yet he felt as if a blasphemy had been committed. His face betrayed his feelings only too clearly.

"I am sorry to disappoint you," said the lady drily.

"You certainly have surprised me," he answered, picking up his hat.

"You are not among our champions, then?"

"I cannot say that the movement has my approval."

"And why?"

"I should much prefer not to discuss it."

"But I am sure you will answer a lady's question."

"Ladies are in danger of losing their privileges when they usurp the place of the other sex. They cannot claim both."

"Why should a woman not earn her bread by her brains?"

Dr. Ripley felt irritated by the quiet manner in which the lady crossquestioned him.

"I should much prefer not to be led into a discussion, Miss Smith."

"Dr. Smith," she interrupted.

"Well, Dr. Smith! But if you insist upon an answer, I must say that I do not think medicine a suitable profession for women and that I have a personal objection to masculine ladies."

It was an exceedingly rude speech, and he was ashamed of it the instant after he had made it. The lady, however, simply raised her eyebrows and smiled.

"It seems to me that you are begging the question," said she. "Of course, if it makes women masculine that would be a considerable deterioration."

It was a neat little counter, and Dr. Ripley, like a pinked fencer, bowed his acknowledgment.

"I must go," said he.

I am sorry that we cannot come to some more friendly conclusion since we are to be neighbours," she remarked.

He bowed again, and took a step towards the door.

"It was a singular coincidence," she continued, "that at the instant that you called I was reading your paper on 'Locomotor Ataxia,' in the *Lancet*.

"Indeed," said he drily.

"I thought it was a very able monograph."

"You are very good."

"But the views which you attribute to Professor Pitres, of Bordeaux, have been repudiated by him."

"I have his pamphlet of 1890," said Dr. Ripley angrily.

"Here is his pamphlet of 1891." She picked it from among a litter of periodicals. "If you have time to glance your eye down this passage—"

Dr. Ripley took it from her and shot rapidly through the paragraph which she indicated. There was no denying that it completely knocked the bottom out of his own article. He threw it down, and with another frigid bow he made for the door. As he took the reins from the groom he glanced round and saw that the lady was standing at her window, and it seemed to him that she was laughing heartily.

All day the memory of this interview haunted him. He felt that he had come very badly out of it. She had showed herself to be his superior on his own pet subject. She had been courteous while he had been rude, self-possessed when he had been angry. And then, above all, there was her presence, her monstrous intrusion to rankle in his mind. A woman doctor had been an abstract thing before, repugnant but distant. Now she was there in actual practice, with a brass plate up just like his own, competing for the same patients. Not that he feared competition, but he objected to this lowering of his ideal of womanhood. She could not be more than thirty, and had a bright, mobile face, too. He thought of her humorous eyes, and of her strong, well-turned chin. It revolted him the more to recall the details of her education. A man, of course, could come through such an ordeal with all his purity, but it was nothing short of shameless in a woman.

But it was not long before he learned that even her competition was a thing to be feared. The novelty of her presence had brought a few curious invalids into her consulting rooms, and, once there, they had been so impressed by the firmness of her manner and by the singular, newfashioned instruments with which she tapped, and peered, and sounded, that it formed the core of their conversation for weeks afterwards. And soon there were tangible proofs of her powers upon the country side. Farmer Eyton, whose callous ulcer had been quietly spreading over his shin for years back under a gentle *regime* of zinc ointment, was painted round with blistering fluid, and found, after three blasphemous nights, that his sore was stimulated into healing. Mrs. Crowder, who had always regarded the birthmark upon her second daughter Eliza as a sign of the indignation of the Creator at a third helping of raspberry tart which she had partaken of during a critical period, learned that, with the help of two galvanic needles, the mischief was not irreparable. In a month Dr. Verrinder Smith was known, and in two she was famous.

Occasionally, Dr. Ripley met her as he drove upon his rounds. She had started a high dogcart, taking the reins herself, with a little tiger behind. When they met he invariably raised his hat with punctilious politeness, but the grim severity of his face showed how formal was the courtesy. In fact, his dislike was rapidly deepening into absolute detestation. "The unsexed woman," was the description of her which he permitted himself to give to those of his patients who still remained staunch. But, indeed, they were a rapidly-decreasing body, and every day his pride was galled by the news of some fresh defection. The lady had somehow impressed the country folk with almost superstitious belief in her power, and from far and near they flocked to her consulting room.

But what galled him most of all was, when she did something which he had pronounced to be impracticable. For all his knowledge he lacked nerve as an operator, and usually sent his worst cases up to London. The lady, however, had no weakness of the sort, and took everything that came in her way. It was agony to him to hear that she was about to straighten little Alec Turner's club foot, and right at the fringe of the rumour came a note from his mother, the rector's wife, asking him if he would be so good as to act as chloroformist. It would be inhumanity to refuse, as there was no other who could take the place, but it was gall and wormwood to his sensitive nature. Yet, in spite of his vexation, he could not but admire the dexterity with which the thing was done. She handled the little wax-like foot so gently, and held the tiny tenotomy knife as an artist holds his pencil. One straight insertion, one snick of a tendon, and it was all over without a stain upon the white towel which lay beneath. He had never seen anything more masterly, and he had the honesty to say so, though her skill increased his dislike of her. The operation spread her fame still further at his expense, and self-preservation was added to his other grounds for detesting her. And this very detestation it was which brought matters to a curious climax.

One winter's night, just as he was rising from his lonely dinner, a groom came riding down from Squire Faircastle's, the richest man in the district, to say that his daughter had scalded her hand, and that medical help was needed on the instant. The coachman had ridden for the lady doctor, for it mattered nothing to the Squire who came as long as it were speedily. Dr. Ripley rushed from his surgery with the determination that she should not effect an entrance into this stronghold of his if hard driving on his part could prevent it. He did not even wait to light his lamps, but sprang into his gig and flew off as fast as hoof could rattle. He lived rather nearer to the Squire's than she did, and was convinced that he could get there well before her.

And so he would but for that whimsical element of chance, which will for ever muddle up the affairs of this world and dumbfound the prophets. Whether it came from the want of his lights, or from his mind being full of the thoughts of his rival, he allowed too little by half a foot in taking the sharp turn upon the Basingstoke road. The empty trap and the frightened horse clattered away into the darkness, while the Squire's groom crawled out of the ditch into which he had been shot. He struck a match, looked down at his groaning companion, and then, after the fashion of rough, strong men when they see what they have not seen before, he was very sick.

The doctor raised himself a little on his elbow in the glint of the match. He caught a glimpse of something white and sharp bristling through his trouser leg half way down the shin.

"Compound!" he groaned. "A three months' job," and fainted.

When he came to himself the groom was gone, for he had scudded off to the Squire's house for help, but a small page was holding a gig-lamp in front of his injured leg, and a woman, with an open case of polished instruments gleaming in the yellow light, was deftly slitting up his trouser with a crooked pair of scissors.

"It's all right, doctor," said she soothingly. "I am so sorry about it. You can have Dr. Horton to-morrow, but I am sure you will allow me to help you to-night. I could hardly believe my eyes when I saw you by the roadside."

"The groom has gone for help," groaned the sufferer.

"When it comes we can move you into the gig. A little more light, John! So! Ah, dear, dear, we shall have laceration unless we reduce this before we move you. Allow me to give you a whiff of chloroform, and I have no doubt that I can secure it sufficiently to—"

Dr. Ripley never heard the end of that sentence. He tried to raise a hand and to murmur something in protest, but a sweet smell was in his nostrils, and a sense of rich peace and lethargy stole over his jangled nerves. Down he sank, through clear, cool water, ever down and down into the green shadows beneath, gently, without effort, while the pleasant chiming of a great belfry rose and fell in his ears. Then he rose again, up and up, and ever up, with a terrible tightness about his temples, until at last he shot out of those green shadows and was in the light once more. Two bright, shining, golden spots gleamed before his dazed eyes. He blinked and blinked before he could give a name to them. They were only the two brass balls at the end posts of his bed, and he was lying in his own little room, with a head like a cannon ball, and a leg like an iron bar. Turning his eyes, he saw the calm face of Dr. Verrinder Smith looking down at him.

"Ah, at last!" said she. "I kept you under all the way home, for I knew how painful the jolting would be. It is in good position now with a strong side splint. I have ordered a morphia draught for you. Shall I tell your groom to ride for Dr. Horton in the morning?"

"I should prefer that you should continue the case," said Dr. Ripley feebly, and then, with a half hysterical laugh,—"You have all the rest of the parish as patients, you know, so you may as well make the thing complete by having me also."

It was not a very gracious speech, but it was a look of pity and not of anger which shone in her eyes as she turned away from his bedside.

Dr. Ripley had a brother, William, who was assistant surgeon at a London hospital, and who was down in Hampshire within a few hours of his hearing of the accident. He raised his brows when he heard the details.

"What! You are pestered with one of those!" he cried.

"I don't know what I should have done without her."

"I've no doubt she's an excellent nurse."

"She knows her work as well as you or I."

"Speak for yourself, James," said the London man with a sniff. "But apart from that, you know that the principle of the thing is all wrong."

"You think there is nothing to be said on the other side?"

"Good heavens! do you?"

"Well, I don't know. It struck me during the night that we may have been a little narrow in our views."

"Nonsense, James. It's all very fine for women to win prizes in the lecture room, but you know as well as I do that they are no use in an emergency. Now I warrant that this woman was all nerves when she was setting your leg. That reminds me that I had better just take a look at it and see that it is all right."

"I would rather that you did not undo it," said the patient.

"I have her assurance that it is all right."

Brother William was deeply shocked.

"Of course, if a woman's assurance is of more value than the opinion of the assistant surgeon of a London hospital, there is nothing more to be said," he remarked.

"I should prefer that you did not touch it," said the patient firmly, and Dr. William went back to London that evening in a huff.

The lady, who had heard of his coming, was much surprised on learning his departure.

"We had a difference upon a point of professional etiquette," said Dr. James, and it was all the explanation he would vouchsafe.

For two long months Dr. Ripley was brought in contact with his rival every day, and he learned many things which he had not known before. She was a charming companion, as well as a most assiduous doctor. Her short presence during the long, weary day was like a flower in a sand waste. What interested him was precisely what interested her, and she could meet him at every point upon equal terms. And yet under all her learning and her firmness ran a sweet, womanly nature, peeping out in her talk, shining in her greenish eyes, showing itself in a thousand subtle ways which the dullest of men could read. And he, though a bit of a prig and a pedant, was by no means dull, and had honesty enough to confess when he was in the wrong.

"I don't know how to apologise to you," he said in his shame-faced fashion one day, when he had progressed so far as to be able to sit in an arm-chair with his leg upon another one; "I feel that I have been quite in the wrong."

"Why, then?"

"Over this woman question. I used to think that a woman must inevitably lose something of her charm if she took up such studies."

"Oh, you don't think they are necessarily unsexed, then?" she cried, with a mischievous smile.

"Please don't recall my idiotic expression."

"I feel so pleased that I should have helped in changing your views. I think that it is the most sincere compliment that I have ever had paid me."

"At any rate, it is the truth," said he, and was happy all night at the remembrance of the flush of pleasure which made her pale face look quite comely for the instant,

For, indeed, he was already far past the stage when he would acknowledge her as the equal of any other woman. Already he could not disguise from himself that she had become the one woman. Her dainty skill, her, gentle touch, her sweet presence, the community of their tastes, had all united to hopelessly upset his previous opinions. It was a dark day for him now when his convalescence allowed her to miss a visit, and darker still that other one which he saw approaching when all occasion for her visits would be at an end. It came round at last, however, and he felt that his whole life's fortune would hang upon the issue of that final interview. He was a direct man by nature, so he laid his hand upon hers as it felt for his pulse, and he asked her if she would be his wife.

"What, and unite the practices?" said she.

He started in pain and anger.

"Surely you do not attribute any such base motive to me!" he cried. "I love you as unselfishly as ever a woman was loved."

"No, I was wrong, it was a foolish speech," said she, moving her chair a little back, and tapping her stethoscope upon her knee. "Forget that I ever said it. I am so sorry to cause you any disappointment, and I appreciate most highly the honour which you do me, but what you ask is quite impossible."

With another woman he might have urged the point, but his instincts told him that it was quite useless with this one. Her tone of voice was conclusive. He said nothing, but leaned back in his chair a stricken man.

"I am so sorry," she said again. "If I had known what was passing in your mind I should have told you earlier that I intended to devote my life entirely to science. There are many women with a capacity for marriage, but few with a taste for biology. I will remain true to my own line, then. I came down here while waiting for an opening in the Paris Physiological Laboratory. I have just heard that there is a vacancy for me there, and so you will be troubled no more by my intrusion upon your practice. I have done you an injustice just as you did me one. I thought you narrow and pedantic, with no good quality. I have learned during your illness to appreciate you better, and the recollection of our friendship will always be a very pleasant one to me."

And so it came about that in a very few weeks there was only one doctor in Hoyland. But folks noticed that the one had aged many years in a few months, that a weary sadness lurked always in the depths of his blue eyes, and that he was less concerned than ever with the eligible young ladies whom chance, or their careful country mammas, placed in his way.

14

Starting Up in Practice

An Introduction to Selections from
Daniel W. Cathell's Book on the Physician Himself

The *Book on the Physician Himself and Things That Concern His Reputation and Success* enjoyed extraordinary popularity when it first appeared in 1881. By 1902 it had run to eleven editions, and revised versions continued to be reissued until 1922. It is now something of a historical curiosity, valuable for the insights it affords into the realities of family practice in the late nineteenth century.

Not much is known about its author, Daniel Webster Cathell (1839–1925) who wrote no other books. He graduated in 1865 from the Long Island Medical College, became a respected practitioner in Baltimore, and an active member of the profession. On the title page of the second (1882) edition he lists the many offices he has held: "Late Professor of Pathology in the College of Physicians and Surgeons of Baltimore; Ex-President of the Medical and Surgical Society; Active Member of the Medical and Surgical Faculty at Maryland; Honorary Member of the Lincoln Philosophical Society, etc., etc." This enumeration of his record can be seen as a tactic to validate his qualifications to write this book on the basis of his extensive experience and honored position.

The Physician Himself is a conduct book to guide aspiring doctors in the behavior necessary to achieve a good reputation and financial success. Cathell may have planned the book to help his own son, William, who was born in 1864 and graduated from the medical school in Baltimore in 1886. It was a difficult time to get started in medicine in the United

States because of the overproduction of doctors as a result of the proliferation of medical schools. Their number increased from 52 in 1850
to 75 in 1870, 100 in 1880, 133 in 1890, and 160 by 1900. The schools
varied enormously in quality so that the mere possession of a medical
degree did not suffice to inspire patients' confidence. Cathell's description of some schools as "doctor-making . . . push-'em-through" colleges
not only expresses his own contempt for the low standards and oppor-
tunism of some places but also indicates the problem of the unevenness
of medical training, a problem examined and remedied by the famous
Flexner Report (1910), which recommended a reduction in the total
number of schools and scrutiny of their curricula. Using another derogatory term, "swarms," Cathell cites the influx of immigrant doctors who
escalate what he plainly sees as a "contest" for patients. A knowledge of
this context is vital for an understanding of Cathell's endeavor: he is
motivated by his awareness of the need to *woo* patients. He openly
addresses the issues of overcrowding in the profession and its consequent
competitiveness (see "Too Many Doctors," the first selection). He cites
categoric figures for the comparative density of physicians per population: 1:3500 in Italy; 1:3000 in Germany; 1:2500 in Austria; 1:1814 in
France; 1:1652 in Great Britain; 1:1193 in Canada; and 1:600 in the
United States. Late-nineteenth-century American physicians were therefore exceptionally insecure and dependent on winning and keeping their
patients' favor.

Under these circumstances, Cathell argues in the opening sentence
of his book, that "it is as necessary for even the most scientific physician
to possess a certain amount of professional tact and business sagacity as
it is for a ship to have a rudder." Dividing medicine into "a greater, or
scientific, side" and "a lesser, or personal, side," he declares that "This
little book is an essay on the lesser, or personal, side" which he regards
as crucial for the attainment of "reputation and success." Cathell makes
the implicit assumption that the budding practitioner has an adequate
command of the scientific side. He urges "judicious and intelligent use
of your scientific instruments of precision,—the stethoscope, the ophthalmoscope, the laryngoscope, the clinical thermometer, the tape, the
microscope." This list shows the great growth in the number of scientific
instruments that had come into common use toward the end of the
century. But Cathell always concentrates on the interpersonal aspects of
medical practice; he points out, for instance, that these instruments "will
not only assist you very materially in diagnosis, but will also aid you
greatly in curing nervous and terrified people, by increasing their
confidence in your armamentarium and ability, and enlisting their sym-

pathetic confidence in your remedial treatment." In other words, the psychological impact of the technological tools is just as important, in Cathell's opinion, as their scientific yield. This argumentation is similar to that in the advertising brochures Martin Arrowsmith receives (see chapter 7, the third selection, "How to Obtain Honor and Riches"). Yet in the early editions Cathell still cautions "that cold logic and rigid mathematics, chemistry, psychology, and other high theoretical attainments, however much addressed abstractly, are not a certain guarantee of popular favor, since they are often attained at the expense of the endearing sentiments, and hence create none of those ties upon which many a successful practitioner depends" (1889, 11). Significantly, in the later editions (1905 onward), revised in cooperation with his son, Cathell eliminated or toned down the earlier warnings against being too scientific. So the successive versions of *The Physician Himself* also function as a barometer of the rising prestige of science in medicine.

Near the outset of the book Cathell offers very concrete advice on the optimal way for the doctor to furnish his office (see the second selection, "The Office"). He deals with the choice of a good location, the design of the name-plate, and particularly the furnishing of the office itself. He is engaging in what would nowadays be called image management. His concept of what is appropriate in an office and what would seem either frivolous or unsuitable gives us an unwittingly humorous insight into what actually went on in medical practice. From this angle *The Physician Himself* represents an ethnographic treasure trove. Likewise, Cathell's injunctions on dress are indirectly a telling commentary on prevailing standards and opinions (see "How to Dress," the third selection). But the emphasis on appearance serves ultimately the same purpose as the desirable office decor, namely to foster a positive impression that will induce greater personal confidence in the doctor and consequently a willingness on patients' part to pay larger bills.

Cathell offers categoric advice about handling patients on both a day-to-day and a long-term basis. He underscores affability as the cardinal quality to attract patients; it has to extend beyond the consulting- or sick-room to casual encounters, say in church or on the street (see the fourth selection, "Affability"). Again the primary emphasis is on impressions and appearances: a "very nice man" will fare infinitely better than a standoffish fellow, no matter how learned he is. Indeed, being "refined and pleasing" in manner ranks before being "sufficiently versed in medicine to discharge his duties correctly" among the traits necessary for climbing the ladder of success. The citation that Cathell includes in the section on dress, "Veneering often outshines the solid wood" (albeit prefaced by "Alas!") aptly summarizes the messages he sends in regard to all the matters that have to be of concern to the novice doctor. And Cathell's rather strange habit of punctuating his opinions by snippets of poetry or proverbs can itself be read as a display of his own refinement. This physician is an educated gentleman, who has a command of literary allusions as an expression of his dignity. However, the quotations are embedded in a vigorous, down-to-earth style that testifies too to the writer's commonsensical grasp on reality.

So Cathell emphasizes that friendliness must always be tempered by respect on both sides; undue familiarity ("Hallo, Doc!") is strongly discouraged (see "Dignity," the fifth selection). In contrast to usage earlier in the century, when doctors were frequently offered refreshments, partly to alleviate the fatigue of their travel, by the end of the century and in a more urban setting Cathell advises against dining or taking tea with patients since sociability tends to foster a familiarity detrimental to the maintenance of the respect and dignity now considered appropriate to the physician's status. The guidelines on affability and dignity suggest the wary course the doctor has to steer between excessive friendliness and the least whiff of arrogance. Toward the close of the century the physician is, by virtue of his special knowledge, his patients' social equal even if he has to maneuver for recognition and struggle for income.

Once the doctor is well established, he has to face another difficulty: that of wisely limiting his practice (see the sixth selection, "Limitation of Practice"). Cathell's primary purpose of protecting the doctor's best interests becomes very apparent here. The barely veiled subtext of this passage is concern for adequate financial compensation: how to achieve a maximum return on a minimum of effort. Cathell counsels prompt rendering of bills, and "weeding out worthless patients" as the best means to reduce the doctor's load. With a realism amounting to cynicism Cathell in effect champions the doctor's welfare over the patient's. From the vantage of "a pecuniary sense" he also discourages attendance on remote cases rather than nearer ones which involve less wear and tear on physician and horse, and more readily produce income.

The tactful collecting of remuneration is a tricky issue, for the physician has to avoid alienating patients by undue pressure, yet needs to be paid, and promptly at that (see "Collecting Fees," the seventh selection). Cathell urges physicians to bear in mind their "own necessities" and their obligations to support their dependents: "you must live by your practice," he sternly admonishes. So the business facet of the doctor's relationship to his patients requires meticulous attention. Speedy rendering of bills is recommended in order to elicit timely payment. Patients still in debt, Cathell comments, are less likely to send for the doctor again for fear of incurring yet another bill. Cathell even offers specific instructions for dealing with various classes of patients: "the prompt-paying, the slow-paying, and the never-paying," and for responding to objections to bills. The financial subtext runs as a repeated theme with variations throughout the *Book on the Physician Himself.* The doctor is still, as in the days of Trollope's *Dr. Thorne* (chapter 2), the employee of the patient who makes direct payment to him. Insurance clubs to defray the costs of burial as well as medical care were being organized among factory workers. But in the middle and upper classes the interaction between the doctor and the patient continued to have a distinct commercial dimension. So the physician, especially at a time of acute competition, is constrained to be pleasing to patients in every possible respect; the appearance of his office, his own self-presentation, and his manner, all have to be geared to the bottom line.

Today's reader will no doubt be struck by Cathell's persistent use of masculine pronouns in referring to the physician, from the title of his book onward. On one occasion he does mention women doctors, and is even sufficiently open-minded to allow cooperation with them if necessary. But it is quite clear from the *Book on the Physician Himself* that the medical profession was still perceived at the turn of the century as an almost exclusively male preserve.

Cathell's manual is an interesting counterpart to texts dating from the middle of the century. It points to continuities as well as differences. The major advance is the range of instruments considered a normal part of a physician's equipment by the 1880s in contrast to the simpler, more subjective modes of examination prevalent fifty or so years before. But in many other respects the resemblance to dilemmas faced earlier on is striking. As in the 1847 *Code of Ethics* of the American Medical Association and in Trollope's *Dr. Thorne,* the physician's position is an ambivalent and difficult one as he has to balance the assertion of his dignified status with his financial dependence on patients. The *Code of Ethics* spells out the ideal behavior on both sides whereas the *Book on the Physician Himself* squarely confronts the practical realities. In giving a glimpse behind the scenes of the facade the doctor has to stage and to maintain, it is specific and at times comical. Thus, although the physician must establish his authority, he is strongly advised to tolerate such home remedies as onions and saffron plasters to the feet if that is what it takes to win and keep the patient's favor.

In the hundred years or so since Cathell's book was a popular manual, the structure of the medical profession has changed radically. The introduction of insurance, intended to make medical care more widely accessible, has also brought a third party into the doctor-patient relationship.

With the recent rise of managed care, insurance companies have assumed enormous power over both doctors and patients in asserting their right to determine the appropriate type and duration of treatment. So doctors now have to placate the insurers as well as satisfying patients. Has the physician's position grown more problematical since Cathell's day? Is managed care the price that has to be paid for the extension of medical care beyond those able to afford it out of their own pockets? In view of the tremendous cost of life-saving high-tech procedures such as organ transplants, does health care have to be rationed? If so, who should make the decisions?

Too Many Doctors

Daniel W. Cathell

There has been of late years a large, annual addition to our already overcrowded profession, and, instead of giving a leisurely education and high cultivation, the superabundant, doctor-making colleges of the United States, with their push-'em-through inducements—small fees, condensed lectures, quizzes, "loading up" from compends, epitomes, *vade mecums* (guide manuals), and *multum in parvo* (abbreviated guide-books), and grinding-clubs, with the few short courses of lectures required—are now manufacturing annually more than five thousand graduates, besides the swarms of medical immigrants representing all nations who reach our shores from abroad, already dubbed M.D., and ready to enter the contest at once. The result is that every city, town, hamlet, and village, every cross-roads, yea, every nook and every corner everywhere in our land can now boast a physician or two; and if it requires a population of 1800 people to support each physician, and if every physician must have a paying clientage of 1000 or 1200 persons to enable him to live and thrive, there are now in every American community more than twice as many physicians as are required by the professional work, and in some sections they are actually fighting for charity cases; and, if the number continues to increase, Heaven only knows what will become of the hindmost.

From Daniel W. Cathell, *Book on the Physician Himself* (Philadelphia: Davis, 1905), p. 45.

The Office

Daniel W. Cathell

A corner house is naturally preferable to one in the middle of a row, since it is convenient for persons coming from all directions, and not only has facilities for constructing an office entrance on the side street, leaving the front door free for family use, but also insures fresh air to the consulting-room, and a good light for examinations, operations, and study. If you board, do so in a genteel house, and in a respectable neighborhood, at or close to your office.

Regarding offices: Try to have a nice, comfortable, cheerful waiting-room, with a recessed front door; also, a good, light, airy, and accessible consulting-room of moderate dimensions, with, if at all convenient, two doors,—one for the entrance and the other for the exit of patients,—for many of those who consult you will prefer to be let out through a passage or private door, and thus escape the gaze and possibly the whispering comments of others in waiting.

Exercise special care in their arrangement, and make them look fresh, neat, and clean outside; and give them a snug, bright, and cosy medical tone inside, neither as full as a wareroom nor as barren as a miser's apartments. Let their essential features show that their occupant is possessed of good breeding and cultivated taste, as well as learning and skill;

From Daniel W. Cathell, *Book on the Physician Himself* (Philadelphia: Davis, 1905), pp. 8–11.

and that they are not a lawyer's consulting-rooms, nor a clergyman's sanctum, nor an instrument-maker's shop, nor a smoking-club's headquarters,—with a vile smell of stale cigars or pipes,—nor a sportsman's rest nor a loafing room for the idle, the dissipated, and the unemployed; nor a family parlor, nor a social meeting-place of any kind; but the offices of an earnest, working, scientific physician, who has a library, takes the journals, and makes full use of the instruments of precision, and the various methods that science has devised for doing different kinds of medical and surgical work, and regards his office as the twin sister to the sick-room.

Take particular care, however, to avoid making a quackish display of instruments and tools, and keep from sight such inappropriate and repulsive objects as catheters, syringes, stomach-pumps, obstetrical forceps, splints, trusses, amputating knives, skeletons, grinning skulls, jars of amputated extremities, tumors, manikins, the unripe fruit of the uterus, etc. Also avoid such chilling or coarse habits as keeping vaginal specula or human bones on your desk for ornaments or paperweights:—

A shivering Raw-Head and Bloody-Bone display.

But while you should make no undue exhibition of books, surgical instruments, etc., it is not unprofessional to have about you—not for display, or designedly made conspicuous, but for ready and actual use— your outfit: microscope, stethoscope, laryngoscope, ophthalmoscope, spirit-lamp, testtubes, reagents for testing specimens, and other modern aids to precision in diagnosis, with the various other scientific instruments you make use of in treatment; also to ornament your office with diplomas, certificates of society membership, potted or cut flowers or growing plants or vines, fine etchings, or photographs of your own professional friends or teachers. A galaxy of small pictures of medical celebrities—Hippocrates, Galen, Harvey, Gross, Pasteur, or whomever else you especially admire—may be grouped on the office walls by the dozens or hundreds. Busts or statues are also in excellent taste, and are interesting to all, also academical prizes, professional relics, keepsakes, mementoes, medals, or anything else that tells of your mental or physical prowess in earlier days, or is especially associated with your medical studies and career. But, unless it be a few artistic ornaments or works of art, it is better to limit such articles to those that relate to you as a student or pertain to you or your vocation as a physician.

A surgical chair, a gynecological table, or both are now seen in almost every office, and in good hands, is apt to pay for itself many times a year.

In buying your office-outfit see that the walls and floors are tastefully covered. Articles of furniture should be few in number, but good, including a small and—if means will admit—handsome book-case, with writing-table and chairs to correspond. Have comfortable chairs for your patients' use, and one so arranged that they may sit in a good light during examination; but beware of stocking yourself with novelties and instruments that will probably go out of fashion or rust or spoil before you will need them. It is prudent not to invest heavily at first, but you must have the necessary every-day instruments which the urgency of certain cases will not give you time to go for when occasion arises for their use, and get others only when you have a use for them. Bear in mind that soft-rubber goods, and soft goods generally, deteriorate in keeping and finally become worthless.

A neat case of well-labeled and well-corked medicines is of great use and not unornamental; so also are dictionaries, encyclopedias, and lexicons for ready reference; also a nonstriking time-piece to notify the time quietly to physician and patient by its tick-tock, tick-tock. Also, find a place for a neat looking-glass, or mirror; but display no miniature museum of sharks' heads, stuffed alligators, tortoise-shells, impaled butterflies, ships, steam-boats, mummies, snakes, fossils, stuffed birds, lizards, crocodiles, tape-worms, devil-fish, ostrich-eggs, hornets' nests, or anything else that will advertise you in any light other than that of a cultivated physician. It will, to the thinking portion of the public, seem very much more appropriate for you, as a physician, to be jubilant over a restored patient or a useful medical discovery than to be ecstatic over a stuffed flying-fish, a rare shell, or an Egyptian mummy. If you have a natural love for such incongruous things, or are a bird- or dog-fancier or a bug-hunter, at least keep the fact private, and keep your specimens out of sight of the public, and endeavor to lead patients to think of you solely as an earnest, scientific physician.

How to Dress

Daniel W. Cathell

A decent respect for the opinion of the world should lead you to keep within the limits of good taste in everything and to practice all that constitutes politeness in dress and deportment. Be neither a fop nor a sloven, but keep yourself neat and tidy, and avoid everything approaching carelessness or neglect. And as you will be judged by your dress and address, do not altogether ignore the fashions of the day, for a due regard to the customs prevailing around you will show your good sense and discretion. Even though the prevailing style of dress or living borders on the absurd or extravagant, it may still be wise to conform to it to a certain extent:—

> Though wrong the mode, comply; more sense is shown
> In wearing others' follies than our own.

You never heard of a swindler, or a confidence-man, or a gambler, or a pseudo-gentleman of any kind, who dressed shabbily or in bad taste:—

> These men's souls are in their clothes.

Such people are all close students of human nature, and, no matter how tarnished in character or how blackened in heart, they too often

---

From Daniel W. Cathell, *Book on the Physician Himself* (Philadelphia: Davis, 1905), pp. 28–30.

manage to hide their deformities as with a veil from all but the few who know their true characters, by assuming the dress and manners of gentlemen. Now, if genteel dress, polished manners, and cultured address can do so much for such unworthy specimens of mankind, how much greater influence must appearance, manners, and a guarded tongue exert for those who are truly gentlemen and members of an honorable profession!

Nevertheless, do not, under any plea, be a leader or patronizer of loud or frivolous fashion, as though your egotism and love of sporty clothes had overshadowed all else; avoid glaring neckties, flashy breastpins, loud watch-seals, brilliant rings, fancy canes, perfumes, attitudinizing, and all other peculiarities in dress or actions that indicate overweening self-conceit, or a desire to be considered a fop of fashion or a butterfly swell:—

Cupid, have mercy!

Fops, dudes, and dandies may be admired at the time for posturing, but they are not usually chosen by discerning persons seeking a guardian for their health.

Even though you be ever so poor, let your garb show genteel poverty, for as a physician your dress, manners, and bearing should all agree with your noble and dignified calling, for neglect of neatness of dress and want of polite manners might cause you to be criticised or shunned. You will sometimes see little Dr. Tact, a vastly inferior man, whose scientific capital is very limited, and cranium comparatively empty, and intellectually near-sighted, who always sat on the back benches at college, and was never accused of having an excess of brains, succeed in getting extensive and lucrative practice, and paying heavy bills for horseshoes, almost entirely by attention to the outer trappings and affability of manner; while Dr. Fullhead, Dr. Betterman, and Dr. Talent, professionally more able and personally more worthy, will have but little need of bell-knobs at their doors, and never learn the cost of carriages and the price of horse-feed, or of bonds and stocks, by reason of defects in these apparently unimportant matters. Alas!—

Veneering often outshines the solid wood.

Clean hands, well-shaved face or neatly-trimmed beard, unsoiled shirt and collar, unimpeachable hat, polished boots, spotless cuffs, well-fitting gloves; fashionable, well-made clothing, of fine texture; cane, sun-umbrella, neat office-jacket, etc.—all relate to personal hygiene—severally indicate gentility and self-respect, and impart to their possessor a pleasurable consciousness of being well dressed and presentable:—

> I am not a handsome man, but my make-up doth lend me an air of respectability.

The majority of people will employ a physician with genteel appearance and manners, of equal or even inferior talent, more readily than a slovenly, rough-bearded one; they will also accord to him more confidence, and expect from and willingly pay to him larger bills.

Affability

Daniel W. Cathell

Physicians are made in the colleges, but tried in the world. Your personality and deportment in the presence of patients will have much to do
with your success. Endeavor to make your address as pleasing as possible
and never omit to return a salute. Blessed is the physician who has the
gift of making friends. A pompous, or cold, or cheerless, or indifferent,
or iceberg-manner toward people, especially those who show a desire for
friendship and good-will, or a studied or sanctimonious isolation of one's
self from them socially:—

> Like a frozen island;

or failure to recognize sick-room and other acquaintances on the streets
and elsewhere, as if from a haughty independence, or as if "they are
inferior and entirely beneath me," or as if:—

> I am resolved on dignity or death,

often gives offense and destroys all warmth toward that physician, and
usually causes their owner to fail to inspire either friendship or confidence;
and a physician who cannot in some way make friends or awaken faith

From Daniel W. Cathell, *Book on the Physician Himself* (Philadelphia: Davis, 1905), p. 62.

in himself cannot fail to fail. The reputation of being a "very nice man" makes friends of everybody, and is, with many, even more potent than skill. To be both affable in manner and skillful in action makes a very strong combination: one that aids in wafting its possessor up to the top wave of professional success and repute. If, moreover, he be refined and pleasing in manner and sufficiently versed in medicine to discharge his duties correctly, his politeness will make him a troop of friends, and will be professionally more effective with many people than the most profound acquaintance with histology, microscopical pathology, and other scientific acquirements.

Dignity

Daniel W. Cathell

Preserve a proper degree of gravity and dignity toward your patients. Frivolous conduct, coarse jokes, horse-play, skylarking, clownish levity, vulgar roughness, unseasonable sportiveness and bar-room familiarity are unprofessional, and tend to breed contempt and scandal. Discourage all attempts of roughs and toughs rudely to address you with a "Hello, Doc!" or by your first name, or in any other way to pass the limit of propriety with you. Show every one proper respect, and exact the same in return. Do not, however, understand us to advocate solemn pomposity, or to condemn good-natured pleasantry. Not so; for, when gentlemanly and in moderation, lightheartedness is often very appropriate, and sometimes actually serves as a tonic to a patient's drooping spirits. If you, happily, possess a becoming earnestness of deportment and sobriety of conversation, and at the same time wear a cheerful mien, it will be both health to yourself and sunshine to the sick.

Avoid dining out with your patients and attending their tea- or card-parties. Eat as seldom as possible at their houses,—only when unavoidably detained there by cases of labor, convulsions, and the like. There is a tendency to conviviality and *abandon* around the festive board that has a leveling effect, and divests the physician of his legitimate prestige. It is far better to cultivate no intimacies and eat a cold repast at home than to occupy the best seat at the table and partake of the most savory viands

From Daniel W. Cathell, *Book on the Physician Himself* (Philadelphia: Davis, 1905), p. 122.

of some patients. Let a physician once unbend himself among certain classes of people, and he risks a complete loss of their professional appreciation and their confidence.

Limitation of Practice

Daniel W. Cathell

Keep your practice down to a number that you can properly attend; this you can do by rendering your bills promptly, weeding out worthless patients, limiting the distances you will go to practice, declining other than desirable obstetrical engagements, increasing your charges, etc. In refusing to take a case at a distance, or one that is likely to involve you as a witness in court contrary to your wish, or declining an obstetrical engagement, if you are "too busy," or have too many previous engagements, assign that as your chief reason, and adhere to it, as it is the least open to criticism and persuasibility of any that can be assigned.

Unless you have the advantage of direct rapid transit, attendance on patients at long distances has a tendency to derange and diminish your nearer practice, for while absent attending a remote call you may lose three nearer ones, and miss all else that may happen during that time. Nor do distant visits, as a rule, pay in a pecuniary sense, but they do work a hardship to both physician and patient. A few far-off patients will waste more time, break down more horseflesh, use up more carriages, harass you more at unseasonable hours, keep you from bed, and expose you to bad weather oftener, and do more to make your life a hard one and to wear you out, than all your near-by practice combined.

From Daniel W. Cathell, *Book on the Physician Himself* (Philadelphia: Davis, 1905), p. 148.

Collecting Fees

Daniel W. Cathell

As a physician you will hold two relations to your patients: first, during sickness you will feel personal interest in them and scientific interest in their afflictions, give them your best skill and attention, employing whatever remedies will be most surely, most safely, and most rapidly beneficial. This must ever be your leading purpose, and to this you should add humane sympathy and commiseration. Later, when, by recovery or death, your interest and skill are no longer required, you will enter upon the second, or business relation, and then, unless poverty forbid, you should demand and secure, in a business-like manner, a just remuneration for your services; for you must be clothed and fed, and must support those dependent upon you, just as other people do; for every man naturally and properly looks to whatever occupation he follows for support. Therefore neither false delicacy nor fear of offending those who owe you fees should be allowed to outweigh your own necessities, break up the business feature of your profession, interfere with your rules in money matters, or prevent your knowing where sentiment ends and business begins. Being human, you must live by your practice, just as the priest lives by the altar, the lawyer by the bar, and all other people by their vocations.

From Daniel W. Cathell, *Book on the Physician Himself* (Philadelphia: Davis, 1905), pp. 335, 338–339, 342–343.

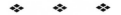

The nearer your financial arrangements approach the cash system, the better it will be for you and your dependents. Frequent accounts are best for the physician. If he renders his bills promptly, it teaches people to look for them and to prepare to pay them, just as they do other family expenses. It is even better to submit to a reduction in bills for prompt payment, than to let them stand and run the risk of losing them through the pay-when-you-please system. Besides, after settling promptly, many patients will feel free to send for you again and make another bill, even in moderate sickness, instead of dallying with home remedies or quack medicines, as they might do if they still owed you.

You should render your bills while they are small, and your services still vividly remembered, not only because gratitude is the most evanescent of all human emotions, but for another reason: if you are neglectful or shamefaced and do not send your bills promptly, it will create the opinion that you do not believe in prompt collecting, or are not dependent upon your practice for a living, or have no need of money; and that, even were they to pay, you would merely throw what they gave you on your pile or put it in bank; or that you do not hold this or that person to your business rule, or are not uneasy about what they owe you. And if you foster a bad system of bill-rendering, a bad system of bill-paying will grow up around you, and great loss will result; because some will die, others will abscond and others become unable to pay:—

Long credits make short friendships and sure losses.

Asking for payment reminds patients that there is still a little human nature left in a man, even if he has become a physician; and that, since you must live, you must have your fees to enable you to do so, and therefore payment is expected.

Besides: The business of the world is now conducted more on the cash system, instead of the old long-credit plan, and you should do your share to:—

Break the legs of the evil custom

that some physicians follow, either through carelessness or to maintain the favor of patients, of waiting six months or a year after rendering services before sending a bill. If a physician attends a person, say in February, and sends his bill in March or April, it seems to the patient like one of his current expenses; it looks as though the physician lived by his practice and has sent his bill as a matter of course, and it is apt to be paid promptly; whereas, if he delays sending it until the following July or January, and then heads it with the semi-apology, "Bills rendered January 1st and July lst," as if an excuse for sending it even then, the debtor will naturally think that the physician has merely audited his books, and sent out this bill with a whole batch of others, more because he has posted the account, than from a special desire for its payment. In this belief he will probably give but little or no attention to it, and let it remain unpaid for months longer, thus delaying its settlement till it becomes an old back debt—which is the hardest kind of a hard bill to pay.

Before you have practiced long you will find that there are three classes of patients: the prompt-paying, the slow-paying, and the never-paying, and that your welfare will depend not upon how much you book, but upon how much you collect, and that if you never insist upon the payment of your fees you can never separate the wheat from the chaff. If you have a business rule, and people know it, they will associate you and your rule together, and be guided thereby. Therefore let patients know, in the early years of your practice, what your rule or system is, or you cannot do so later in life. When a new family employs you, render your bill as soon after the services as ordinary courtesy will allow, especially if there has been a previous attendant who was a careless or indifferent collector or no collector at all. Send it somewhat as a test, and if there be any objection to you consequent on the prompt presentation of your bill, or because you want your fee, the sooner you arrive at an understanding of each other, or part company, the better for you, and the less apt will you be to surround yourself with a horde of worthless patients.

Some physicians have more tact in getting fees than others, and, curiously enough, there are people who will pay one physician but will not pay another, there being certain ones with whom they desire to stand well and others for whose opinions they do not care. Try to be in the former class with all persons of doubtful integrity.

When patients ask you how much their bills are, or how much they are indebted for office-consultations, operations, etc., always reply, with courteous promptness and decision, "one dollar," "ten dollars," or whatever else the amount way be, large or small; and if you be careful to avoid prefacing or following this reply with other words, and neither hesitate nor stammer, most people will, in the embarrassment of the moment, proceed to pay you without objection; whereas if you show uncertainty or add more words it will weaken your claim in their minds, or impress them with the belief that you have no fixed charge, and furnish them with a pretext to show surprise and to ask for a reduction. When one does demur at the amount, show your amazement, and be prepared at once to defend or explain the justice of the charge.

Further Historical and Literary Readings

Historical

Abel-Smith, Brian. *The Hospitals 1800–1940*. Cambridge: Cambridge Univ. Press, 1964. A history of British hospitals.

Akerknecht, Erwin H. *A Short History of Medicine*. 1955. Baltimore: Johns Hopkins Univ. Press, rev. ed., 1982. A good reference book, packed with information, but rather dry.

Allsop, Giulielma Fell. *History of the Women's College of Philadelphia, Pennsylvania, 1850–1950*. Philadelphia: Lippincott, 1950. A case study of one important women's medical college.

Apple, Rima D., ed. *Women, Health, and Medicine in America: A Historical Handbook*. New York: Garland, 1990. A useful source book.

Bell, E. Moberly. *Storming the Citadel: The Rise of the Woman Doctor*. London: Constable, 1953. A fine account of women in medicine in Great Britain.

Bernard, Claude. *Introduction à l'étude de la médecine expérimentale*, ed. Paul F. Cranefield. New York: Science History Publications/USA, 1976; Introduction to the Study of Experimental Medicine, trans. Henry Copley Greene. 1865. Reprint, New York: Macmillan, 1957. The key work that envisaged medicine as an essentially scientific endeavor.

Blackwell, Elizabeth. *Pioneer Work in Opening the Medical Profession to Women*. 1895. Reprint, New York: Schocken, 1977.

————. *Essays in Medical Sociology*. 1902. Reprint, New York: Arno Press and *New York Times,* 1972. Expositions of "maternal" medicine as the appropriate alternative mode for women physicians.

Blake, Catriona. *The Charge of the Parasols: Women's Entry into the Medical Profession*. London: Free Press, 1990. A succinct account of women physicians in Great Britian.

Bynum, W. F. "Hospital, Disease and Community: The London Fever Hospital, 1801–50." In *Healing and History,* edited by Charles E. Rosenberg. New York: Dawson Science History Publications, 1979, 91–115. A detailed study of one hospital's role in the early part of the century.

Cartwright, Frederick A. *A Social History of Medicine*. New York: Longman, 1977. Focuses on the social aspects of medicine in the community.

Cunningham, Andrew, and Perry Williams, eds. *The Laboratory Revolution in Medicine*. Cambridge: Cambridge Univ. Press, 1992. A collection of articles documenting laboratory discoveries.

Drachman, Virginia. *Hospital with a Heart: Women Doctors and the Paradox of Separatism at the New England Hospital, 1862–1969*. Ithaca: Cornell Univ. Press, 1984. Examines the debates among women doctors about the proper way for them to run a hospital.

Ehrenreich, Barbara, and Deirdre English. *Complaints and Disorders: The Sexual Politics of Sickness*. Old Westbury, N.Y.: Feminist Press, 1973. A feminist view of the doctor-patient relationship.

Foucault, Michel. *The Birth of the Clinic*. Trans. A. M. Sheridan Smith. New York: Vintage, 1975. An imaginative interpretation of the history of the hospital filtered through the author's theories.

French, Roger, and Andrew Wear, eds. *British Medicine in an Age of Reform*. London: Routledge, 1991. A collection of illuminating articles on various facets of nineteenth-century British medicine.

Furst, Lilian R. *Between Doctors and Patients: The Changing Balance of Power.* Charlottesville: Univ. of Virginia Press, 1998. Medical history 1830 to the present in and through literary texts.

————, ed. *Women Healers and Physicians: Climbing a Long Hill*. Lexington: Univ. of Kentucky Press, 1997. Twelve essays (six on the nineteenth century) exploring diverse aspects of women's medical activity in various countries.

Guthrie, Douglas. *Janus in the Doorway*. Springfield, Ill.: Charles C. Thomas, 1963. The development of the microscope, 208–21.

Hooker, Worthington. *Physician and Patient; or, A Partial View of the Mutual Duties, Relations and Interests of the Medical Profession and the Community*. 1849. Reprint, New York: Arno Press and *New York*

Times, 1972. The mid-century vision of the physician as the patient's (and the family's) "confidential friend."

Jacobi, Mary Putnam. *Mary Putnam Jacobi, M.D.: Pathfinder in Medicine.* 1882. Reprint, New York: Putnam, 1925. The ideas of the American sponsor of scientific medicine as suited to women.

Jex-Blake, Sophia. *Medical Women.* 1886. Reprint, New York: Source Books, 1970. The British pioneering woman doctor's pleas in favor of admitting women to the medical profession.

Jones, Anne Hudson, ed. *Images of Nurses: Perspectives from History, Art, and Literature.* Philadelphia: Univ. of Pennsylvania Press, 1988. A collection of essays.

Kett, Joseph. *The Formation of the American Medical Profession: The Role of Institutions 1780–1860.* New Haven: Yale Univ. Press, 1968. An analysis of the impact of institutions on the formation of American medical practice.

King, Lester S. *Transformations in American Medicine: From Benjamin Rush to William Osler.* Baltimore: Johns Hopkins Univ. Press, 1991. A survey of early American medical history.

Kruif, Paul de. *Microbe Hunters.* New York: Harcourt Brace (1926) 1983. A popular, highly readable account of twelve microbe researchers spanning from the seventeenth to the early twentieth century.

Maulitz, Russell. "Channel Crossing: The Lure of French Pathology for English Medical Students 1816–36." *Bulletin of the History of Medicine* 55 (1981): 475–96. Documents the attraction of French medical advances early in the century.

Morantz-Sanchez, Regina Markell. *Science and Sympathy: Women Physicians in American Medicine.* New York: Oxford Univ. Press, 1985. Comprehensive history of women in American medicine.

Murphy, Lamar Riley. *Enter the Physician: The Transformation of Domestic Medicine, 1760–1860.* Tuscaloosa: Univ. of Alabama Press, 1991. The growing role of physicians (as against home remedies) in the development of American medicine in the later eighteenth and early nineteenth century.

Newman, Charles. *The Evolution of Medical Education in the Nineteenth Century.* New York: Oxford Univ. Press, 1957. Traces the changes in medical training.

Nuland, Sherwin B. *Doctors: The Biography of Medicine.* New York: Vintage, 1988. A selective history of fifteen major turning-points in the development of medicine from Hippocrates to the twentieth century through a series of studies of innovators in their fields at their time; includes a lively chapter on Laënnec and the stethoscope.

Parry, Noel, and José Parry. *The Rise of the Medical Profession*. London: Croom Helm, 1976. Concentrates on Great Britain.

Peterson, Jeanne M. *The Medical Profession in Mid-Victorian London*. Berkeley: Univ. of California Press, 1978. The organization and practices of nineteenth-century British medicine.

Porter, Roy. *The Greatest Benefit to Mankind: A Medical History of Humanity*. New York: Norton, 1998. Recent, comprehensive survey of the history of medicine from antiquity to today.

Reiser, Stanley Joel. *Medicine and the Reign of Technology*. Cambridge: Cambridge Univ. Press, 1978. Technological advances, especially in instrumentation.

Rosenberg, Charles E. *The Care of Strangers*. New York: Basic Books, 1987. A history of hospitals in the United States.

———. *The Cholera Years: The United States in 1832, 1849, and 1866*. Chicago: Univ. of Chicago Press, (1962) 1987. The response to successive epidemics.

Rosenberg, Charles E., and Morris J. Vogel, eds. *The Therapeutic Revolution: Essays in the Social History of American Medicine*. Philadelphia: Univ. of Pennsylvania Press, 1979. A collection of essays on progress in therapeutics.

Rosenberg, Charles E., and Janet Golden, eds. *Framing Disease*. New Brunswick: Rutgers Univ. Press, 1992. A collection of articles on diverse factors affecting the history of medicine.

Rothstein, William G. *American Physicians in the Nineteenth Century*. Baltimore: Johns Hopkins Univ. Press, 1972. A history of mainstream, male physicians.

Shorter, Edward. *Bedside Manners: The Troubled Relations between Doctors and Patients*. New York: Simon & Schuster, 1985. Argues that doctor-patient relations have by their very nature always been fraught with difficulties.

Shryock, Richard Harrison. *The Development of Modern Medicine: An Interpretation of the Social and Scientific Factors Involved*. 1936. Reprint, Madison: Univ. of Wisconsin Press, 1979. A wide-ranging history of medicine.

Starr, Paul. *The Social Transformation of American Medicine*. New York: Basic Books, 1987. A history of American medicine from a sociological angle.

Vogel, Morris. *The Invention of the Modern Hospital*. Chicago: Univ. of Chicago Press, 1980. A case study of the history of the Massachusetts General Hospital in Boston.

Waddington, Ivan. *The Medical Profession in the Industrial Revolution.* Dublin: Gill and Macmillan Humanities Press, 1984. The effect of industrialization on the structure of medical practice.

Walsh, Mary Roth. *"Doctors Wanted: No Women Need Apply" Sexual Barriers in the Medical Profession, 1835–1875.* New Haven: Yale Univ. Press, 1977. The history of discrimination against women in medicine in the United States.

Warner, John Harley. *The Therapeutic Perspective: Medical Practice, Knowledge, and Identity in America.* Cambridge: Harvard Univ. Press, 1986. A scholarly examination of the progress of American medicine in its many ramifications.

Woodham-Smith, Cecil. *Florence Nightingale.* New York: Atheneum (1951) 1983. Still the best biuography of the pioneer of professional nursing.

Literary

Alcott, Louisa May. *Hospital Sketches.* 1863. Records her experiences as a nurse during the Civil War.

———. *Jo's Boys.* 1886. Includes a young woman who plans to be a doctor.

Alexander, G. G. *Dr. Victoria: A Picture from the Period.* 1881. A melodramatic and rather sentimental picture of an early British woman doctor.

Anon. *Dr. Edith Romney.* 1883. A long romantic novel about the vicissitudes of a British woman doctor's career.

Bailin, Miriam. *The Sickroom in Victorian Fiction: The Art of Being Ill.* New York: Cambridge Univ. Press, 1994. The rituals of illness through patients' and nurses' perceptions.

Balzac, Honoré de. *Médecin de campagne* (Country Doctor). 1833. A novel about a rural practitioner who cares lovingly for his patients and carries out hygienic and social reforms.

Biasin, Gian-Paolo. *Literary Diseases: Theme and Metaphor in the Italian Novel.* Austin: Univ. of Texas Press, 1975. Changing interpretations of disease in Italian literature.

Cline, C. L. "Qualifications of the Medical Practitioners in Middlemarch." In *Nineteenth-Century Perspectives: Essays in Honor of Lionel Stevenson,* edited by Clyde D. L. Ryals. Durham, N.C.: Duke Univ. Press, 1974, 271–81. Analysis of the various medical men in Eliot's novel.

Eliot, George. "Janet's Repentance," *Scenes from Clerical Life*. 1858. Reprint, New York: Oxford Univ. Press, 1988, 167–301. Contrasts an old style family doctor who grasps problems through long-standing knowledge of his patients with a progressive practitioner who uses a stethoscope but lacks empathy.

Fontane, Theodor. *Effi Briest*. 1895. Trans. Douglas Parmée. Harmondsworth: Penguin, 1956. The physician as a family friend with psychological insight.

Gaskell, Elizabeth. *Wives and Daughters*. 1866. The life and work of a British country surgeon in the late 1820s.

Holmes, Oliver Wendell. *Elsie Venner*. 1861. Dr. Kittredge, who is able through his tactful presence and understanding to soothe Elsie.

Howells, William Dean. *Dr. Breen's Practice*. 1881. A critical portrayal of a diffident woman doctor.

James, Henry. *The Bostonians*. 1886. The scientifically advanced Dr. Mary Prance can also show kindness to a dying patient.

Meyer, Annie Nathan. *Helen Brent, M.D.* 1891. A superwoman surgeon, president of a women's medical college, advocate of scientific medicine.

Phelps, Elizabeth Stuart. *Dr. Zay*. 1882. A romance about a highly competent and successful woman practicing in Maine about 1880.

Reade, Charles. *A Woman-Hater*. 1877. An aggressive woman doctor's struggle for admission to the profession, based on British history.

Rothfield, Lawrence. *Vital Signs: Medical Realism in Nineteenth-Century Fiction*. Princeton: Princeton Univ. Press, 1992. A study of the use of medicalized language in nineteenth-century fiction.

Travers, Graham. *Mona Maclean: Medical Student*. 1893. The determined young woman who succeeds in both studying medicine and marrying a fellow practitioner.

Turgenev, Ivan. *Fathers and Sons*. 1862. The old folkloric and the new scientific medicine in Russia in mid-century.

Twain, Mark, and Charles Warner Dudley. *The Gilded Age*. 1873. An early portrayal of a young woman who goes into medicine but ends up in marriage.

Zola, Emile. *Dr. Pascal*. 1893. A late-nineteenth-century French doctor who combines small-town practice with research in pursuit of the elixir of life.

Index

311